Love heals. *The Daniel Plan* will allow you to begin healing at the deepest levels because it is based on the power of science *and* the power of love. Profoundly inspiring and highly recommended!

— DEAN ORNISH, M.D., Founder and President, Preventive Medicine Research Institute; Clinical Professor of Medicine, University of California, San Francisco; author, *The Spectrum*

FAITH + FOOD + FITNESS + FOCUS + FRIENDS

# THE DANIEL PLAN

## 40 Days *to a* HEALTHIER LIFE

RICK WARREN D.MIN.
DANIEL AMEN M.D.
MARK HYMAN M.D.

*with Sean Foy and Dee Eastman*

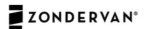

This book is dedicated to you.
Our hope and prayer is that this book inspires you
to begin your journey toward health —
and that you experience a whole new level of wellness.
In the process we pray you feel God's presence, his power,
and his purpose for your life.

*Dear friend, I pray that you may enjoy good health
and that all may go well with you,
even as your soul is getting along well (3 John 2).*

## DISCLAIMER

*The Daniel Plan* offers health, fitness, and nutritional information and is for educational purposes only. This book is intended to supplement, not replace, the professional medical advice, diagnosis, or treatment of health conditions from a trained health professional. Please consult your physician or other healthcare professional before beginning or changing any health or fitness program to make sure that it is appropriate for your needs — especially if you are pregnant or have a family history of any medical concerns, illnesses, or risks.

If you have any concerns or questions about your health, you should always consult with a physician or other healthcare professional. Stop exercising immediately if you experience faintness, dizziness, pain, or shortness of breath at any time. Please do not disregard, avoid, or delay obtaining medical or health-related advice from your healthcare professional because of something you may have read in this guide.

# Contents

# Bible Versions

# Chapter 1

# How It All Began
## PASTOR RICK WARREN

*Wow! Everybody's FAT!*

That shocking thought kept reverberating in my mind one bright spring day as I was baptizing 827 adults.

I'll admit it wasn't a very spiritual thought for a pastor to have, especially while baptizing! But I was getting tired, since our church baptizes the way Jesus was baptized in the Jordan River — by lowering people under the water, then lifting them back up.

That day, based on the average weight of Americans, I lifted more than 145,000 pounds!

I had read plenty of articles about the growing epidemic of obesity, diabetes, and heart disease in America, but that day I actually *felt the weight* of America's health problem in a dramatic way.

While my first thought was that everyone I baptized was overweight, my second thought was more personal and pointed:

*But I'm fat too! I'm as out of shape as everyone else is!*

In that moment of clarity, I realized the terrible example I was giving with my own health. How could I expect my congregation to take better care of their bodies if I was such a poor model? I had ignored my own growing problem for thirty years.

Let me explain:

I grew up in a family that didn't drink alcohol or smoke, but all food — no matter how unhealthy it might be — was considered okay. And growing up, much of my life centered around food.

Every memory of my childhood, both good and bad, was connected to food. When we were happy, we celebrated by eating. When we were sad, we consoled ourselves with comfort food. If I had a difficult day as a child, the antidote was cookies and milk or a piece of fresh pie.

Living on five acres in the country, my dad grew a huge vegetable garden, my mom loved to cook, and we all loved to eat. Eating was our entertainment, and we had huge meals every night. In fact, our handmade fourteen-foot dining table made of a single four-inch slab of redwood was the largest piece of furniture in our house. It dominated our home, and our family life revolved around the meals we shared together.

Blessed with good health, a high metabolism, and an active life, I could eat everything I wanted and as much as I wanted and never gain a pound. When I married Kay, I was as thin as a flagpole even though I rarely exercised and ate junk food constantly. I paid no attention to my health.

Then, in 1980, at age twenty-five, I became the founding pastor of Saddleback Church in Southern California. As the church rapidly grew to thousands of members, I worked long days, ate meals on the run, and spent hours sitting while leading meetings, counseling people, and studying for sermons. I began adding a few pounds every year, but because my energy remained high and I didn't care much about appearance, I ignored my growing health problem. By 2010, I was severely overweight.

Ironically, over the past decade I had sent nearly 21,000 of our church members overseas to 196 countries to serve the sick and the poor through a program we developed called the P.E.A.C.E. plan. The C of the P.E.A.C.E. stands for "Care for the sick," and our members had compassionately cared for the health of others around the world who were suffering from poor nutrition, poor water, malaria, and HIV/AIDS. But I ignored my own declining health and that of my own members.

That baptism was my wake-up call to the health issues in my life and in the lives of those in our congregation. I knew drastic changes were needed, so I began educating myself about preventative health. What I learned shocked me:

- For the first time in history, as many people are suffering from the result of *too much* food as malnutrition. While millions of people suffer from not having enough to eat, millions are struggling with the effects of being overweight.[1]
- Seven in ten Americans are overweight.[2]
- Diabetes, heart disease, and other "lifestyle-based diseases" now kill more people than infectious diseases worldwide.[3]

The next Sunday, I stood before my congregation and made this public confession:

Friends, I've been a poor steward of my health and a terrible example for you. While we've been helping many around the world, I've ignored the problem here at home.

So today I am publicly repenting, and I ask for your forgiveness! God expects us to take care of the bodies he has given us, but I have not done that. Now, I've only gained two to three pounds a year, but I have been your pastor for thirty years. So I need to lose ninety pounds! Do any of you want to join me in getting healthy?

The audience responded with sustained applause.

Honestly, I expected that maybe a couple hundred people would join me in my quest to get healthy, so I was overwhelmed when more than 12,000 people signed up in the first few weeks! Now I needed a plan. It had to be simple, inexpensive, and scalable. Since I was preaching that day about a man in the Bible named Daniel who refused to eat junk food and challenged a king to a health contest, I named the program The Daniel Plan.

Since I knew nothing about getting healthy, I recruited three nationally known doctors — Dr. Daniel Amen, Dr. Mark Hyman, and Dr. Mehmet Oz — to coach me in getting healthy and help me design

The Daniel Plan to be used in our church. All three doctors graciously volunteered their expertise and time for free because they care about our health.

Over the first year of The Daniel Plan, Saddleback members collectively lost more than 250,000 pounds! But even more important, we learned insights, developed skills, and established habits for a lifetime of healthy living. The Daniel Plan is far more than a diet. It is a lifestyle program based on biblical principles and five essential components: Food, Fitness, Focus, Faith, and Friends. These last two components — faith and friends — are what I call *the secret sauce* that makes The Daniel Plan so effective. When you have *God and a group* helping you, you now have far more than willpower helping you make positive changes, and you are far more likely to stay consistent.

Let me be clear: There is no magic pill, no quick fix, no instant formula, and no shortcut that will make you healthy overnight. You must make wise choices *every day*. You will likely have setbacks. I have! In fact, as I write these words, I am recovering from a recent setback. My family experienced a tragic loss that was devastating to all of us. In my grief, I didn't sleep much, and that left me exhausted, both emotionally and physically. Overwhelmed by sorrow and fatigue, I stopped making healthy choices and began to add unwanted weight. All those pounds I had lost kept finding me! But as anyone in recovery will tell you, setbacks are part of the process in long-term change. Rather than beat myself up, I simply asked God and my friends to help me get back on track.

The plan you will read about in this book is really quite simple. Dedicate your body to God. Ask for his help, and get involved in a small group of some kind that will support you on your journey. Then start making healthy choices — such as replacing donuts with fresh fruit and making exercise a part of your daily routine. Make whole foods a regular part of your diet. Live a more active lifestyle. Get more sleep. Cut down on your stress. It's not rocket science. It's just good, common sense. After all, God expects you to use the brain he gave you.

Many diets and fitness plans use guilt as a motivation, but that never works in the long run. You can guilt yourself into doing anything short-term, but the change will last only as long as the guilt (or fear) does. In contrast, The Daniel Plan is built with *love* as the motivation: Experiencing God's unconditional love for you, learning to love him back, learning to love whom God made you to be, and learning to give and receive love from others in a small group setting.

The Bible says, "Love never gives up, never loses faith, is always hopeful, and endures through every circumstance" (1 Corinthians 13:7 NLT). It is love — not fear, not guilt, and not peer pressure — that causes us to keep going when we feel like giving up.

The Bible also tells us that lasting change begins with *committing your body* to God. Romans 12:1 – 2 says, " ... *give your bodies to God. ...* Let them be a living and holy sacrifice — the kind he will find acceptable. This is truly the way to worship him. Don't copy the behavior and customs of this world, but *let God transform you into a new person by changing the way you think*" (NLT, emphasis added). Notice the strong mind-body connection in this verse. Two thousand years after this verse was written, we now know that not only do our minds affect our bodies, but also our bodies affect our minds.

What you do with your body sets the tone for everything else. Physical health influences your mental health, your spiritual health, your emotional health, your relational health, and even your financial health. How many times have you read a book, heard a message, or attended an event that motivated you to make some change, but then you didn't have the physical energy to do it? Instead, you laid down on your couch and watched TV.

A major motivation for me to be physically healthy is that I want the energy and alertness to make other changes in my life. My guess is that you too have other areas of your life you would like to improve. So we are going to begin by raising your energy level, since you can't do anything without a body! We are going to start at the most basic level of your life: your physical health.

## WHAT DOES GOD SAY ABOUT YOUR BODY?

The Christian family I grew up in attended church services every week. I have listened to thousands of sermons on what God has to say about our souls, our minds, our wills, and our emotions. But not once had I ever heard an entire sermon on God's view of our bodies. The subject was completely ignored. This is why most people still have no theology of health. While our culture is obsessed with physical beauty and sexy bodies, many believers ignore their bodies as if they don't matter. But they do.

God has a lot to say about the importance of the body he gave you. It is talked about through the Bible. But for the sake of brevity, let me show you just one chapter of the Bible, 1 Corinthians 6:12 – 20:

> "I have the right to do anything," you say — but not everything is beneficial. "I have the right to do anything" — but I will not be mastered by anything. You say, "Food for the stomach and the stomach for food, and God will destroy them both." The body, however, is not meant for sexual immorality but for the Lord, and the Lord for the body. By his power God raised the Lord from the dead, and he will raise us also. Do you not know that your bodies are members of Christ himself? Shall I then take the members of Christ and unite them with a prostitute? Never! . . .
>
> Flee from sexual immorality. All other sins a person commits are outside the body, but whoever sins sexually, sins against their own body. Do you not know that your bodies are temples of the Holy Spirit, who is in you, whom you have received from God? You are not your own; you were bought at a price. Therefore honor God with your bodies.

Wow! This is definitely an in-your-face, tell-it-like-it-is, no-holds-barred description of what God considers to be the right and wrong use of our bodies. In this and other passages of Scripture we learn five radical truths about our bodies that run counterculturally to everything you hear today.

*1. My body belongs to God.* It is his property, not mine. I don't own it, God does. He created my body, and he expects me to use it the way he intended for it to be used. Now we naturally rebel against this idea. Our culture teaches us, "My body is mine to do whatever I want to with it." But God says, "No, you're wrong. It's not your body, because you didn't create it. I made it, and I loaned it to you to live in while I put you on earth, and I expect you to take care of my creation."

The fact is, everything you can see on earth was created by God. He made it, and he owns it. What you think you own is really on loan. The Bible says, "The body … is not meant for sexual immorality but for the Lord, and the Lord for the body" (1 Corinthians 6:13).

Today we make the same common mistake Greek philosophers did thousands of years ago. Aristotle, Socrates, and Plato believed in dualism,[4] which included the idea that your mind (or spirit) is important, but your body isn't important spiritually. They devalued the body. In fact, some Greek philosophers taught that your body is evil, so it really didn't matter if you messed it up.

The Bible tells us the exact opposite. Your body is holy because God made it, and everything God makes has a purpose. We are to bring glory to God with our bodies, so we can't compartmentalize our lives and think that we can divorce our bodies and live as if only our spirit matters. God owns your body!

*2. Jesus paid for my body when he died for me on the cross.* As we saw earlier, 1 Corinthians 6:19 – 20 tells us that our bodies have been bought!

Millions of TV viewers love watching *American Pickers* and *Pawn Stars* because it's fun to guess how much old items are worth. The owners often think something they own is more valuable than it really is. But the reality is that something is only worth whatever someone is willing to pay for it! You may think your house is worth more, but it's really only worth what a buyer is willing to pay for it.

God has never made a person he didn't love. If you want to know how valuable your life is to God, just look at the cross. With his arms outstretched, nailed to the cross, Jesus was saying, "This is how valuable you are to me. I love you *this* much! I'd rather die than live without you." You are priceless.

Now, if you are worth dying for, don't you think God wants you to take better care of yourself? If you bought a million-dollar race horse, would you feed it junk food and keep it up all night? Of course not! You would protect your investment. The fact is, Jesus has made an investment in you. He paid for your life with his life, and he expects you to take care of his investment.

**3. *God's Spirit lives in my body.*** When you say yes to God, accepting by faith what Jesus did for you and trusting his grace and forgiveness to save you, then God puts his Spirit inside you as a guarantee of your salvation. The Bible says it like this: "Do you not know that your bodies are temples of the Holy Spirit, who is in you, whom you have received from God?" (1 Corinthians 6:19).

When God puts his Spirit inside you, your body becomes a temple of God, a residence for his love. So let me ask you this: If you saw someone vandalizing or damaging a temple dedicated to God, wouldn't you consider that a crime? Of course! But you abuse and vandalize God's temple, your body, when you deprive it of rest and sleep, overeat, put too much stress on it, and fail to take care of it.

**4. *God expects me to take care of my body.*** I am not the owner of my body, but I am the caretaker, or manager, of it. The word for *manager* in the Bible is *steward.* Taking care of my body is an issue of spiritual stewardship. In fact, God tells me that one day I will have to give an account for how well I managed everything he gave to me, including my body. I will stand before God and have to answer the question, "What did you do with what I gave you?"

In *The Purpose Driven Life* I explain how your life on earth is a test, a trust, and a temporary assignment. This life is preparation for our next life, which will last forever in eternity. God is testing you on earth to see what he can trust you with in eternity. He is watching how you use your time, your money, your talents, your opportunities, your mind, and yes, even your body. Are you making the most of what you've been given? God isn't going to evaluate you on the basis of the bodies he gave to other people, but he *will* judge what you did with what you have been given.

*5. God will resurrect my body after I die.* God never wastes anything. He gets the maximum use out of all he creates. Right now you are living in the 1.0 version of your body. You will get the 2.0 version of your body in heaven. The Bible says, "By his power God raised the Lord from the dead, and he will raise us also" (1 Corinthians 6:14).

We don't really know what our resurrected bodies will be like, but we do have a few clues. We know that after Jesus came from the grave, he walked around Jerusalem for forty days in a resurrected body. He was seen multiple times by many different groups of people, including one event where more than 500 people saw and talked with him. So we know that other people will still recognize you in the new 2.0 version of your body in heaven, but there will be one major difference: in heaven your body will be perfect, with no blemishes, no broken parts, no wounds, and no pain.

Did you notice the phrase *by his power* in that last Bible verse? This is what makes The Daniel Plan different from other approaches. It is built on trusting in God's power to help you change, not merely your own willpower. Let's be honest. Willpower works for a few weeks, or maybe a month or two at best. This is why New Year's resolutions never last. Trying to change by willpower alone is exhausting. You can keep it up for a while, but it feels unnatural and stressful to force yourself to be different simply on the basis of willpower.

In The Daniel Plan you will learn the power of prayer, the power of faith, the power of letting God's Spirit refocus your thoughts, the power of fellowship and community in a supportive small group, and most of all, the power of God's Spirit inside you, helping you to make the changes God wants you to make and you want to make.

## HABITS ARE THE KEY TO YOUR SUCCESS

Making big and lasting changes in our lives is never easy — whether it's changes in the way we relate to others, the way we manage our time, the way we use our money, the way we do our work, or the way we treat our bodies. Whenever we want to improve or change something, we usually start out with great enthusiasm and hopeful expectations, but over time, those feelings fade, and so does our resolve. That is why the key to long-lasting success is to develop *habits* — new, positive habits that replace our self-defeating behaviors. The Bible speaks of *"putting off our old self and putting on a new self,"* which includes our habits (see Ephesians 4:22, 24).

Our habits control our lives. We shape our habits; then our habits shape us. If I asked you to make a list of all your bad habits, you would quickly identify them. You already know what they are, and you know that they aren't helpful. In fact, many are harmful. So why haven't you replaced them? What makes breaking bad habits and creating new ones so difficult? Here are four of the most common reasons:

- **You've had your unhealthy habits for a long time, so you're comfortable with them.** Regardless of whether you are overweight or anorexic, whether you overeat or have any kind of eating disorder, whether you are out of shape or don't have enough energy, you didn't get that way overnight. It was likely a long, slow decline in your health. Many of your adult habits were developed in your childhood. Some of your unhealthy habits may have been survival tactics for unmet emotional and spiritual needs that you experienced early in life. Other habits you developed out of fear. Some habits are developed to soothe negative emotions such as loneliness, anxiety, depression, or feeling unloved.

- **You identify with your unhealthy habits.** Anytime you hear someone say, "I'm always late" or "I'm a worrier" or "I can never resist a dessert," that person is identifying himself or herself with a bad habit. We often confuse our identity with our habits, but the truth is, habits can be changed! Habits are things you *do*. They are not *who you are*! You *have* weaknesses, but you are not your weaknesses. You are a unique creation of God, flawed by your nature and choices, yet deeply loved by God. No man or woman will ever love you as much as God does. His love for you is not dependent on your habits.

- **Your unhealthy habits have a payoff.** In the long run they cause pain, but in the short term they seem easier and more rewarding. And whatever gets rewarded gets repeated. The addicting taste of junk food, the short-term high from carbohydrates, or the pleasure of loafing around instead of exercising gives immediate gratification. We want to feel good *now,* not later.

  God warns of this when he said, "There is pleasure in sin for a short time" (see Hebrews 11:25). Most of the social problems we see in our culture today are the direct result of our unwillingness to delay gratification. To overcome this, you must see the greater payoff and rewards of making healthy choices.

- **You have an enemy who wants to discourage you.** Not only do you have to fight against your natural inclinations, but Satan — whom the Bible calls *the Deceiver* and *the Accuser* — is actively working against you every moment of your day. Since Satan cannot hurt God directly, he tries to hurt God's children. Satan does not want you living a healthy life because that honors God. So he is constantly suggesting negative thoughts to keep you stuck. He loves to plant seeds of doubt in your mind: "Who do you think you are? You're never going to change! You have never been able to change in the past. What makes you think this will be any different? It's hopeless, and you're hopeless. So don't even try!" (In the chapter on Focus, we will have more to say about replacing negative thoughts.)

With these four elements working against us, it is no wonder that most attempts by people to develop healthy habits end in failure. Again, you need more than just good intentions and willpower to change. You need God's plan for change.

## FIVE ELEMENTS FOR LASTING CHANGE

The Daniel Plan is based on five elements for lasting change that are found in John 8, Ephesians 4, and many other Bible passages:

**1. Lasting change requires building your life on the truth.**

One of the most famous statements by Jesus is in John 8:31 – 32: "If you continue to obey my teaching, you are truly my followers. Then you will know the truth, and the truth will make you free" (NCV). Jesus promises that the truth will make you free. But first, the truth is likely to make you miserable! We don't like to face the truth about ourselves, our weaknesses, our bad habits, and especially our motivations. But until you face the truth about *why* you do what you do and get to the root of your habits, change is likely to be shallow and short-lived.

Too often, popular diet fads offer fast formulas, easy pills, and secret cures that supposedly will melt the fat away. By contrast, The Daniel Plan helps you to face the truth about yourself and your relationship to God, to food, to your purpose in life, and to other people. If you are looking for a quick fix, you can set this book down now. But if you want to build an authentically healthy life based on the truth of God, and you're willing to be honest with God, yourself, and a few trusted friends, keep reading.

Nothing will change permanently until you dig down to the bedrock of truth about your life and God's purpose for it. This book is an introduction to get you started on the right pathway, but the journey will take the rest of your life.

**2. Lasting change requires making wise choices.**

Everyone *wants* to be healthy, but very few people *choose* to be healthy. It takes more than desire or a dream to get healthy … it takes a *decision*. You won't change until you *choose* to change. You don't get healthy by accident. It's intentional. It's a choice. Actually, it's a lifetime of choices, but it begins with a decision.

As a pastor I have met many people who were praying for God to heal illnesses and sicknesses that could easily be reversed if they simply made healthier choices. Why should God heal you of an obesity-related illness if you have no intention of changing the choices that led to it? God is waiting for you to start making healthy choices. So if you have been waiting for a sign, this is it!

As you make more and more healthy choices, you will begin to

change: "Get rid of your old self, which made you live as you used to
— the old self that was being destroyed by its deceitful desires. Your
hearts and minds must be made completely new, and you must put on
the new self, which is created in God's likeness" (Ephesians 4:22 – 24
GNT).

## Whose Slave Are You?

Years ago, Bob Dylan sang, "You're gonna have to serve somebody. It may be the Devil or it may be the Lord." In today's
culture that encourages irresponsibility, I counsel many people
who have become slaves to their own desires. Every time you
make a bad choice, it becomes harder to make a good one.
Romans 6:16 says, "Don't you realize that you become the
slave of whatever you choose to obey? You can be a slave
to sin, which leads to death, or you can choose to obey God,
which leads to righteous living" (NLT).

Fortunately, God offers you his power to make healthy choices.
"For God is working in you, giving you the desire and the power to
do what pleases him" (Philippians 2:13 NLT). As you begin to follow
The Daniel Plan, you will see how God has a part and you have a part
in your physical health and your spiritual maturity.

You do what you can do, and God does what only he can do.

### 3. Lasting change requires new ways of thinking.

The way you think determines the way you feel, and the way you feel
determines the way you act. If you want to change how you act, you
must begin by changing the way you think. Your thoughts are the
autopilot of your life.

Romans 12:2 says, "Don't copy the behavior and customs of this
world, but let God transform you into a new person by changing
the way you think. Then you will learn to know God's will for you,
which is good and pleasing and perfect" (NLT). The biblical word

for changing your mind is "repentance." To repent is to make a mental U-turn. I choose to focus my thoughts in a completely different direction. This new mind-set creates new emotions, which give me motivation to change.

Let me ask you a personal question: What old ways of thinking do you need to change? Where do you need to *repent*? Have you held on to some self-destructive ideas about food, about your body, about sex, or about work that have harmed your health? To get healthy, you'll need to *repent* of unhealthy choices. You'll need to think differently about your body — and every other area of your life too. Philippians 2:5 says, "Have the same mind-set as Christ Jesus." The way you do this is by filling your mind with the Bible, God's truth.

In The Daniel Plan, you will learn some new thinking skills, such as learning to replace negative thoughts rather than resisting them. Whatever you resist, persists. The more you fight a feeling, the more it controls you. The secret of victory over any temptation is simply to change the channel of your mind. Refocus your attention on something else, and the temptation immediately loses its power over you.

**4. Lasting change requires God's Spirit in your life.**
I have already mentioned that you need God's power, not just willpower, to change.

God's Holy Spirit helps us break free from bad habits, compulsions, and addictions. Since he offers to help, it would be foolish to not take advantage of it. Galatians 5:18 asks, "Why don't you choose to be led by the Spirit and so escape the erratic compulsions of a law-dominated existence?" (MSG).

The more I allow God's Spirit to guide and empower me, the more he grows positive character qualities in my life to replace my bad habits. The Bible calls these qualities the *Fruit of the Spirit*. Galatians 5:22 – 23 gives a list of them: "But the fruit of the Spirit is love, joy, peace, forbearance, kindness, goodness, faithfulness, gentleness and self-control." Note that last quality: self-control. You already know how important that one is and the damage that happens when you don't have it. But what most people don't know is that the secret of self-control is to allow ourselves to be Spirit-controlled.

This is the exact opposite of what most people think. Ask someone on the street, "What do you think of when I use the phrase 'Spirit-filled' or 'Spirit-controlled'?" and typically people will describe someone acting out of control. But the Bible says that the more I allow God's Spirit to direct and guide me, the more self-controlled I become! As the apostle Paul said, "For I can do everything through Christ, who gives me strength" (Philippians 4:13 NLT). Only a Bible-based program like The Daniel Plan can offer this promise.

### 5. Lasting change requires honest community.

Here's the reality: Some of your habits and patterns and behaviors are so deeply ingrained that you will never be able to uproot and replace them on your own. You have probably tried to change many times and have failed to maintain the changes. If you could change these tough areas by yourself, you would have already done so. But some habits are so strong, we must team-tackle them together.

Actually, this is a good thing, because it forces us to recognize our need for each other. It's part of God's plan. We were created to live in community. We are designed by God for relationships. The very first thing God said to mankind was "It is not good for the man to be alone" (Genesis 2:18). God hates loneliness. So he made us to need each other.

The deepest changes in your life will only happen as you open up to a few trusted friends who will support you and check up on you. You don't need a legalistic schoolmaster, but you do need some friends who will meet with you regularly as a small group. At Saddleback Church we have more than 32,000 people meeting weekly in more than 7,000 small groups, so I speak with confidence in telling you that if you are serious about making lasting changes in your life, the best and most effective way to do it is with the support of others. At Saddleback Church, when 12,000 people lost more than 250,000 pounds, we discovered that those connected to a small group lost twice as much as those who tried to do the program on their own.

In another chapter you learn some specific ways that a small group can assist you in your journey to health by encouraging you, praying for you, supporting you, and giving you feedback.

The Bible is filled with verses on the importance of community. Hebrews 10:25 says, "Let us not give up meeting together, as some are in the habit of doing, but let us encourage one another" (NIV 1984). Galatians 6:2 says, "By helping each other with your troubles, you truly obey the law of Christ" (NCV).

> And Solomon said, "Two people are better off than one, for they can help each other succeed. If one person falls, the other can reach out and help. But someone who falls alone is in real trouble.... A person standing alone can be attacked and defeated, but two can stand back-to-back and conquer. Three are even better, for a triple-braided cord is not easily broken" (Ecclesiastes 4:9 – 12 NLT).

You don't need a lot of people to form your Daniel Plan small group. You can begin with just two or three people. Jesus said, "For where two or three gather in my name, there am I with them" (Matthew 18:20). This is part of "the faith factor" of The Daniel Plan. Jesus will be with you.

As you read through these chapters, you will realize that The Daniel Plan is not complicated, but rather simple and straightforward: You assess your current health and then dedicate your body to God. You ask for God's help. You gather a few friends and form a weekly support group. You begin to make healthy choices that will become habits as you reinforce them. Finally, you expect God to empower you to be consistent, claiming the promise of Philippians 1:6: "Being confident of this, that he who began a good work in you will carry it on to completion until the day of Christ Jesus."

I am proud of you for wanting to be healthier, and I hope you will join thousands of us who have used The Daniel Plan as a tool to change what we feared could never change. This is your moment! There is no telling what God might want to do through you as you gain more energy, think more clearly, feel more confident, and grow physically stronger and more flexible.

I will be praying for you, specifically the words of 3 John 2: "Dear friend, I pray that you may enjoy good health and that all may go well with you, even as your soul is getting along well."

As you begin The Daniel Plan, I would love to hear from you about what happens in your life, in your small group, and in your church. You can email me at *PastorRick@saddleback.com*, connect with me on Twitter (@RickWarren), Facebook (PastorRickWarren), or LinkedIn (PastorRickWarren). And please register at The Daniel Plan website (*danielplan.com*) so you will receive *Daily Hope*, my free daily devotional, and other helpful resources. Welcome to the journey!

## Reflect and Take a Step ...

Are you ready to start your journey to a healthier life? Is it time to make some changes? Go ahead; make the commitment to yourself and God. We have lots of support in the coming chapters that will give you the foundation you need to succeed.

Set up your FREE profile. Go to *danielplan.com* now.

# Chapter 2

# The Essentials

*"Love the Lord your God with all your heart and with all your soul and with all your strength and with all your mind"; and, "Love your neighbor as yourself" (Luke 10:27).*

Steven Komanapalli weighed more than 320 pounds when he started The Daniel Plan through Saddleback Church. His cholesterol was high. His triglycerides were close to 400 mg/dL (normal being around 150 mg/dL). He was pre-diabetic and on multiple medications.

As Steven reveals, "My Daniel Plan journey started when my wife and I started talking about the arrival of our first child and the plans and decisions we would make as parents and as a couple. One of the things that came up was our longevity. She said to me, 'If you die early, man, I'm going to miss you. But if you die of something that was preventable, I'll be really disappointed that you didn't do everything you possibly could to be here for me and for your daughter.' Well, she only had to say that once to get my attention."

Steven took it seriously, and whatever The Daniel Plan doctors and Pastor Warren recommended, Steven did it. He examined his faith. He asked his men's group to support him. He started planning his days around healthy foods. He found active games that interested him to move his body. More than two years later, Steven is down 80 pounds, and his health numbers are improved. He is even taking fewer medications. He is still "doing" The Daniel Plan because it has changed his life.

Hopefully, Steven's story inspires you. We have told you why health is so important, and we have told you part of Steven's story to show you how doable it is. Now we want to show you five areas of your life that work together to affect your health — for good or for bad. The Daniel Plan is based on five *Essentials*: faith, food, fitness, focus, and friends.

The Essentials are a pathway to much more than improved physical health. Each of the Essentials holds up your life, enlivens your body, enriches your mind, and fills your heart. Integrating these can lead to a whole, healthy life that helps you love fully, serve joyfully, and ultimately live out your calling at your best. We want to wake up and be able to give our highest gifts. And we want that for you too.

Pastor Warren dives into your spiritual health and walks with you as you build that foundation. Dr. Hyman tells you everything you need to know about the power of food to affect your mind and body. Once you see how good the right foods can be for you, we hope it will inspire new eating habits that you enjoy.

Exercise physiologist Sean Foy removes the roadblocks that keep you from exercising. He shows you how much fun moving your body is and all the benefits that come from it. Dr. Amen helps you turn your brain into the powerful tool God made it to be by showing you how to boost its physical health, renew your mind, and fulfill your purpose.

The powerful synergy of these Essentials with the support of friends brings you more than any one essential alone. The prophet Daniel didn't simply choose to eat healthier; he made that choice based on his faith, with a clear focus and the support of his friends. So it's no wonder that he was in better shape and health than the others in the king's court.

## THE FAITH ESSENTIAL

Here is a very frank question: Do you quit on your faith every time you hit a bump? Do you say, "Forget it, God. I just can't do this one hundred percent of the time, so what's the use?" No! We know our faith relies on God. He's the one who builds it and sustains it.

God gives us the grace and power to have a relationship with him. His Word instructs us on running this race of faith. God's power is the key to any transformational change in our lives, including our health. He wants us to plug into that power so that we can live and move the way he intended.

If you really believed God's power was behind you, energizing and sustaining you, what would hold you back?

The Daniel Plan starts with faith, because spiritual health gives you a foundation for building habits and perspectives for health in any area. As Pastor Warren mentioned in chapter 1, faith is part of the secret of The Daniel Plan. You may have tried a dozen diets and a dozen exercise programs. But health is about more than a program. Health comes from recognizing and using God's power in your life and treating your body and mind with the care that he intended.

Where God guides, he provides. What he calls you to do, he equips you to do. He doesn't need your strength and willpower, but he does need your commitment. He wants you to live an abundant life that includes a vibrant faith, a vibrant body, and a vibrant mind. But you must rely on Jesus.

For too many of us, unhealthy choices have left us without the mental, physical, or spiritual energy to embrace what God has put us on this planet to do. Some of you think, "It's too late for me. I'd do it if I were younger, but I've wasted my opportunity. I'm woefully out of shape now. I'll never get to where I need to be." But it's never too late.

> "There has never been the slightest doubt in my mind that the God who started this great work in you would keep at it and bring it to a flourishing finish on the very day Christ Jesus appears" (Philippians 1:6 MSG).

Consider your faith — it's always changing, always growing, always being challenged. Sometimes you step forward. Sometimes you step back. But you know faith is a life-long race. Hebrews 12:1 – 2 says, "Let us run with perseverance the race marked out for us, fixing our eyes on Jesus, the pioneer and perfecter of faith."

You have to believe you can get healthy even if you can't see it yet. Hebrews 11:1 says, "Now faith is confidence in what we hope for and assurance about what we do not see." Faith is visualizing the future in advance. It is seeing the future in the present. Every great achievement began when somebody saw it in advance. When President John F. Kennedy issued the challenge to put a man on the moon, the technology hadn't even been invented to do it.

The same is true when it comes to getting healthy. You look in the mirror and believe that, with God's help, you'll get healthy even though the person staring back at you is exhausted, stressed, out of shape, or overweight.

## A Great Gift

"With faith, I embraced the change [of The Daniel Plan lifestyle] and took it head-on. I didn't know where I would land spiritually, but I knew I had to stay close to God. I can recall the day when I felt the Spirit telling me that the vessel God made of me was no longer to be in my control. He was breaking it down against my stubborn will, for my own good. He was about to make a new creation, something adorned in His fashion, that would somehow inspire others. I had to embrace it, and I knew deep down that this would impact my life in more ways than I could imagine."

—Matthew Burstein

You have to keep going even when you want to quit. Holocaust survivor Corrie Ten Boom said, "If you look at the world, you'll be distressed. If you look within, you'll be depressed. But if you look at Christ, you'll be at rest." It all depends on where your focus is; where you bring your mind's attention determines how you feel.

There will be tough days on this journey to healthy living. If you start the habit of turning to God in tough times, then when you face challenges with food, fitness, or focus, you will be in the habit of turning to him for help. God's grace is always there, even when you are tired or tempted.

You have to believe that God has your best in mind even when you can't see what he is doing. Throughout The Daniel Plan, we do our best to explain why — both biblically and scientifically — we are making certain recommendations. But in the end, it will come down to your relationship with God and the health of your faith.

Abraham is a classic example of obeying when he didn't understand. He was about seventy-five years old, and God asked him to give up all his security (Hebrews 11:8). Remember Abraham's faith when you start to wonder things such as:

- "How healthy will I get on this plan?"
- "How long is it going to take?"
- "How will I know when I get there?"

You have to trust God even when you don't get what you want. We all know from personal experience that faith doesn't exempt us from problems. It's easy to trust God when life is going well and we feel strong. But faith develops in the valleys. When our dreams shatter and we feel helpless, that's when we have to believe in God's power and presence. So if you have ever been in a valley and your faith was tested, then you know exactly how to face the lows on the journey of health: trust God.

Faith can virtually be regarded as a verb. It is active and not passive. It is something you do. Decision making is a faith-building activity. Use your muscles of faith to build your physical muscles.

God has given you a mission in life, and only you can fulfill it. Are you going to let your health stand in the way? Are you going to be able to face your Savior at the end of your life and say, "I finished the race. I did what YOU put me on earth to do. I didn't get tired and worn out. I gave Jesus everything, including my physical health"? That's what we hope you can say. So we want to help you build your faith by plugging into God's power and asking him to open your eyes to his view of your life. It will transform you from the inside out.

## THE FOOD ESSENTIAL

What do you really know about food? You know what you like. You know what you don't like. You know what gets your kids excited to eat. Believe it or not, food is much more than your mealtime sustenance. Food can reinvigorate your health, reconnect families, restore vibrant communities, improve the economy, improve the health of the environment, reduce pollution, and even help our kids get better grades and avoid eating disorders, obesity, and drug abuse.

> "So whether you eat or drink or whatever you do, do it all for the glory of God" (1 Corinthians 10:31).

How many of us have ever considered that food can heal? This is the biggest scientific discovery since the germ theory of disease and antibiotics: food is medicine. Food is the most powerful drug on the planet. It can improve the expression of thousands of genes, balance dozens of hormones, and optimize tens of thousands of protein networks. It can cure most chronic diseases, and it works faster, better, and cheaper than any drug — and all the side effects are good ones.

Food contains messages, instructions, and information that tell your body what to do every moment to increase vitality or create disease. Every bite you take is a powerful opportunity to create healing

### How Bad Is It?

One in two Americans suffer from some chronic disease.[1] Heart disease; diabetes; cancer; dementia; autoimmune diseases; allergies; acid reflux; irritable bowels; neurological problems; depression; attention deficit hyperactivity disorder; thyroid, hormonal, and menstrual problems; skin problems including eczema, psoriasis, acne, and more. We spend almost $3 trillion a year in our health care system, and almost 80 percent of that is for chronic lifestyle preventable and reversible disease.[2]

or infirmity. Real, whole food that comes from the earth — food that was created by God — heals, while industrial-processed food created in factories by man harms.

Unfortunately, many of us don't eat food anymore. We eat factory-made, industrially produced food-like substances. This should make us stop and think. Should we really be putting that stuff into our bodies?

### Dump the Junk

The National Institutes of Health spends $800 million a year trying to discover the cause of obesity.[3] Could it be the 29 pounds of French fries, 23 pounds of pizza, 24 pounds of ice cream, 53 gallons of soda, 24 pounds of artificial sweeteners, 2.7 pounds of salt, 90,000 milligrams of caffeine consumed every year by the average American?[4]

We think of these foods as "convenience" foods. For a long time, the invention of jarred, canned, and packaged foods seemed like a great idea for easier cooking and convenient, on-the-go meals. But now we have discovered that this convenience has led to depression, obesity, fatigue, and the surge of people taking multiple medications for lifestyle diseases such as heart disease, depression, and acid reflux. How convenient is that?

The good news is that a life of abundance and vitality is right around the corner. In fact, it is right in our own kitchens. It is time to get back into our kitchens and take back our health. We have been convinced that it is time-consuming, expensive, and difficult to eat well. We are here to tell you that enjoying real, fresh, whole food is easy, inexpensive, and most important, delicious.

The Daniel Plan is rooted in a very simple principle: Take the junk out and let the abundance in. The choice is yours. We don't want to focus on what you can't eat (although we will educate and caution you about certain food substances) as much as on what you can include — delicious whole foods full of extraordinary flavor, delightful textures, and hidden surprises. Our philosophy is that if it was grown on a plant, eat it. If it was made in a plant, leave it on the shelf.

> Our philosophy is that if it was grown on a plant, eat it. If it was made in a plant, leave it on the shelf.

Yes, we encourage eating lots and lots of vegetables. Our theory about vegetables is this: if you hate them, you've never had them prepared properly. They were canned, overcooked, boiled, deep-fried, or highly processed and tasteless mush. Just think of overcooked Brussels sprouts or mushy canned green beans. Those definitely don't sound or taste very appetizing.

As Dr. Hyman says, "Cooking is a revolutionary act." We have unfortunately abdicated the essential act of cooking — the unique act that makes us human — to the food industry. We have become food consumers, not food producers or makers. We have outsourced our cooking to corporations. We need to bring the cooking back home. Cooking can be fun, freeing, and simple.

The Daniel Plan is designed to cut cravings, satisfy your appetite, and teach you to listen to your body. You may not believe it yet, but your body will naturally start rejecting the junk — the sugary, processed, and refined foods — and you will begin to crave real food.

You will be invited to eat natural foods that bring vitality and energy to your body and mind. As you slowly introduce real whole fresh food, your body will respond automatically and heal, and chronic symptoms will fade into memory. The Daniel Plan introduces you to a whole new world of fresh fruits and vegetables, beans, whole grains, nuts, seeds, eggs, chicken, fish, lean or naturally raised animal products, and spices. The Daniel Plan gives you a clear, goof-proof plan.

We are deeply concerned about our fat and sick nation, about our children's and your children's future. The best medicine for this ailment is something so simple, so easy, so healing, so affordable, and so accessible to almost everyone: cooking real, whole food in the home with your family and friends.

## THE FITNESS ESSENTIAL

Be honest — what do you think of when you hear the word *fitness*?

Most of us understand that to have a fit, healthy, energetic, and abundant life, we need to exercise. But the reality is, most of us don't. In fact, more than 70 percent of us are not exercising regularly enough to maintain our health. It's not because of a lack of information or education. For years we have been encouraged, pushed, and prodded by medical doctors, fitness professionals, and government agencies that for a fit and healthy life, we need to exercise.

Like food, exercise works better than medicine. So what keeps us from taking our regular dose? If we are honest, for many of us, exercise isn't something we look forward to doing. It's not on the top of our to-do list.

These sentiments may sound familiar:

"Who has the time or energy to exercise regularly?"

"I've tried to exercise before, but I just can't seem to make it a habit."

"Exercise isn't a lot of fun; it's really a lot of work!"

"When I exercise, all I feel is pain!"

Most of us will admit that exercising regularly is difficult with an already crammed, busy, and hectic schedule. And for those of us who begin to move, we will quit after just a few weeks. If you find yourself in these statistics, you are not alone — but more importantly, we have great news for you.

We would like to share with you a different approach to fitness — one that will help you actually look forward to exercise instead of dreading it. It's a proven method for moving your body, helping you to realize God's purpose, pleasure, and plan for your fitness and health.

Unlike fitness regimens offered in popular health and fitness books, infomercials, DVDs, or gym classes, exercise physiologist Foy will show you how to maximize and enjoy your fitness experience so you can become what we call *Daniel Strong*.

The prophet Daniel was a strong man. In body, mind, heart, and

**Power Walker**

In her fifties, Patti Kaminski never would have dreamed that she would become a fitness fanatic. "I have gone from hardly being able to walk to my front door [when I weighed 110 pounds more than I do today] to walking six miles in the hills every Saturday. Once a month I walk eight miles." She even found a personal trainer and loves going to the gym. "Now my trainer is my workout buddy and my new unofficial adopted son. I love every minute! I have energy like crazy, memory improvement (steel trap), and a complete change on my outlook on life."

spirit, he found his power, purpose, and strength in devotion to God. No matter where he was or what he was doing, he lived with passion and singular focus: to honor God in all he did. Whether he found himself in the comfort of the king's court or in the darkness of a lions' den, Daniel was ready and able to follow God with commitment, devotion, and strength rarely seen. He was fit to serve, whenever, wherever, under extreme difficulty, and in any and all circumstances. He was Daniel strong. But like all of us, he wasn't born with this strength. Rather, he nurtured it by following God's plan and design for his life.

Daniel was recognized early for his potential and was chosen as a young boy to serve the king of Babylon. He diligently trained physically, intellectually, relationally, and spiritually with the purpose to be the best he could possibly be. With a strong body, a strong mind, a strong character, and most of all a strong faith, Daniel honored God in all he did — and you can too.

Another Daniel strong man was Eric Liddell, a man celebrated and remembered from Olympic history for a race he never ran. It was the 100-meter qualifying heat of the 1924 Olympic games hosted in Paris, France. Liddell was the favorite in the event and was expected to take home the Olympic Gold medal for his country. But his qualifying race was scheduled on a Sunday, the day he observed as the Sabbath. To the shock and dismay of the press and the racing world, Liddell, a devout Christian, withdrew from the race, desiring to honor God above others' expectations, great opposition, and his own personal gain.

A few days later, Liddell focused his attention on a race that was not one of his better events, the 400 meters. Since he was racing against a field of world record-setting competitors, very little was expected of Liddell in this event. Yet, not only did he win the 400-meter race, but he also broke the existing world record with a time of 47.6 seconds, a record that would stand for years.

## Exercise Medicine

Exercise is the best strategy to:

- Increase energy
- Improve muscular strength, tone, and endurance
- Make you happier, reducing stress, anxiety, and depression
- Look and feel years younger
- Manage weight and decrease body fat
- Increase productivity
- Stimulate creativity
- Sharpen focus
- Promote restful sleep
- Enhance intimacy and relationships
- Strengthen bones
- Make you smarter
- Enhance immune function
- Increase joint mobility
- Improve posture
- Treat and prevent more than forty chronic diseases

Need we say more?

Liddell is known for saying, "When I run, I feel God's pleasure." This quote embodies the man, servant, and athlete Eric Liddell. It also captures the very essence of what fitness in The Daniel Plan is all about.

But we don't have to be Olympic athletes — or even train like one — to capture the profound lesson that Eric Liddell's life demonstrated. Liddell discovered that his love of running, training, and exercising not only made his body strong and healthy, but also gave him great satisfaction and joy and prepared him to be in the best shape he could be for the rest of his life.

Leading health and wellness organizations such as the American College of Sports Medicine have discovered that moving your body even just a little bit on a regular basis impacts not only your physical health, but also your intellectual, emotional, social, financial, and spiritual health.

Like Daniel and Eric Liddell, we are designed to move. When we are fit, our bodies, minds, and relationships work better, and we have the potential, resilience, and strength to be all we were designed to be.

Wherever you are at with fitness — even if you have never exercised on a regular basis — The Daniel Plan will help you find a personal fitness strategy that you will enjoy. We will help you discover what moves you so that you can build and strengthen the body God gave you.

## THE FOCUS ESSENTIAL

You can have solid faith, healthy food choices, and plenty of exercise and still sabotage your health. The potential saboteur? Your brain. Your mental health is vital for your overall health. Negative thoughts, positive thoughts, or lack of thought can consume you. Depending on which one consumes the most of your mind, you could make or break your health before you even get started. Whatever gets the most of your mind's attention will direct many other areas of your life.

When your brain works right, you work right. When your brain is healthy, your ability to focus increases and you make better decisions.

## Change Your Mind

"Whatever is true, whatever is noble, whatever is right, whatever is pure, whatever is lovely, whatever is admirable — if anything is excellent or praiseworthy — think about such things" (Philippians 4:8). Part of staying focused is being able to develop mastery over the quality of your thoughts. Thoughts lie — they lie a lot. It is often your uninvestigated thoughts that drive depression, anxiety, fear, and overeating that derail progress toward better health.

So many distractions compete for your attention, so it is important to renew your mind and focus on God's plan and priorities for your life.

Ultimately, the health of your brain heavily influences the quality of your decisions and your ability to maintain focus. Your brain is involved in everything you do. Modern-day neuroscience clearly tells us that when your brain works right, you tend to be happier, physically healthier, and more thoughtful, because you make better decisions. (Decision making is a brain function.)

A patient who was a mixed martial arts (MMA) fighter came to see Dr. Amen. One might imagine MMA is not good for the brain. This patient had been fighting competitively for more than five years and struggled with his focus, temper, and mood. Using the Essentials of The Daniel Plan — which included more deeply connecting with his purpose, changing his diet, engaging in non-brain-damaging exercise, using some simple supplements to enhance brain function, and connecting with friends — this patient was able to show remarkable improvement.

One of the most important parts of the Focus Essential is to know your motivation, or why you must get healthy. Without an underlying clear sense of motivation, it is much harder to stay the course in good times and hard ones. But once you know why you care, why you must be healthy, your motivation literally provides the fuel for staying focused. Ask yourself why you must be healthy. Is it to live in God's will? To have greater health and mental clarity? Or to be a great role model for someone you love?

Every time you have a thought, your brain releases chemicals. Negative, angry, and hopeless thoughts produce negative chemicals that make your body and mind feel bad; by contrast, positive, happy, and hopeful thoughts produce a completely different set of chemicals that help you feel relaxed, happy, and in control of your impulses. We will explain several ways your mind distorts the truth. Knowing how to talk back to your negative thoughts is critical to being able to focus on the truth in God's Word and helping you live in the fullness of mental and physical health that God wants for you.

In a similar way to disciplining your mind to have accurate, honest thoughts, it is also important to bring your attention each day to those things for which you are grateful. Modern medical research reveals that when you consistently focus on your blessings and what you are grateful for each day, it has positive effects on your physical and mental health. For example, psychologist Martin Seligman from the University of Pennsylvania found that when people wrote down three things they were grateful for each day, within three weeks it significantly increased their level of happiness.[5] As you will see, gratitude even helps your brain work better.

## Losing More Than Pounds

Laura, a fifty-three-year-old project manager, had struggled with her weight for many years. She had tried diet after diet without lasting success. Learning how to focus on gratitude, correct her negative thought patterns, and learn from mistakes rather than beat herself up, together with the elements of faith, food, fitness, and friends made a huge long-term difference for her. She lost forty-three pounds over six months and became dedicated to a new way of living instead of a fad diet.

Often, attempts to improve your health or life fall flat or end too soon because your willpower is hard to build. You know that your willpower must rest on the power of God, but it also grows stronger with a clear mind and self-control. Think about how often you try to avoid something bad for you but fail because you cannot control your impulses. It's frustrating, isn't it? So, what if you could learn the two most important words in the English language when it comes to your health: *then what*.

- *Then what* will happen if I eat this?
- *Then what* will happen if I say this impulsive thing to my wife?
- *Then what* will happen if I stay up at night on the computer and don't get good sleep for tomorrow?

Keeping these two words at the top of your mind and engaging in the right habits, such as getting enough sleep and eating right, will make a dramatic difference in your mental and physical health, which in turn will help your friendships and your connection with God.

Clear focus and a healthy mind don't preclude failure on this journey. Failure is a part of everyone's journey. But it is your attitude toward failure that will determine your ultimate success. Focus and a healthy mind can help you have the right attitude toward failure. We are telling you now to expect both ups and downs on your journey toward better health. There will be highlights and setbacks.

Failure does not have to defeat or derail you. It can actually increase your chances of ultimate success. The Daniel Plan encourages you to turn bad days into good information and to study your failures. Learning from your mistakes helps to prevent them in the future.

One of Dr. Amen's favorite exercises to help people get and stay healthy for a lifetime is called The Fork in the Road.

Vividly imagine a fork in the road with two paths:

To the left, imagine a future of pain. If you don't care about your brain and body and just keep doing what you've always done, what will your life be like in a year ... in five years ... in ten years? Imagine your body continuing to get old and all that goes with that ... brain fog, tiredness, depression, memory loss, and physical illness.

To the right, imagine a future of health. If you care about your body, which is a gift from God, and do The Daniel Plan, what will your life be like in forty days, in a year ... in five years ... in ten years? Imagine your body and spirit getting healthier and all that goes with that ... mental clarity, better energy, a brighter mood, great memory, a trimmer and healthier body, healthier skin, and a healthier brain.

Boost your brain health, and you will boost all your other efforts for a healthier life.

## THE FRIENDS ESSENTIAL

For many of you, this isn't the first time you have tried to get your health under control. The secret sauce — friends — brings it all together.

When it comes to your health, every *body* needs a *buddy*. After all, God created the universe in such a way that we need each other. In fact, the New Testament uses the phrase *one another* over and over. It says love one another, encourage one another, serve one another, support one another. The word "support" literally means to increase one another's potential.

Doesn't that sound like something you want? You already have it in some way. You may have a prayer circle that supports your spiritual walk. You may meet with a dinner club in which everyone finds joy in cooking. You may be part of a moms or dads group where you all talk about the daily challenges of raising your kids. You have friends who support you.

Now consider what your journey toward whole health would be like if you did it in community. Research shows that people getting healthy together lose twice as much weight as those who do it alone.[6] That success dramatically increases when you are connected with others, receiving constant encouragement to stay focused and motivated toward your goals.

Friends and faith set apart The Daniel Plan as a lifestyle that is attainable and maintainable. Diet and nutrition books can give you the nuts and bolts, but only the mutual support of others can increase your results and sustain them.

The wisest man in the world, King Solomon, knew it: "Two are better than one" (Ecclesiastes 4:9).

The prophet Daniel understood this principle too. He didn't make his commitment to God's ways and healthy choices by himself. He did it with three friends. The four of them — together — were much stronger than any of them could have been alone.

God never meant for you to go through life solo, and that includes your journey toward better health. Whether you join with a few neighbors, ask parents of your kids' friends, start a group at the office, sign up for a church small group, or gather your family, find a few others to start The Daniel Plan with you. Social connections are critical. When you are surrounded by people who have the same values, goals, and health habits, you are going to progress farther than you could on your own.

> Learn more practical tips about getting healthy through the five Essentials. Invite some friends to do *The Daniel Plan DVD Study and Study Guide* together. Go to *danielplan.com* to register your group and get started.

For example, when you're facing a tough situation, who do you turn to? Your friends or family, those who know you best, those who will pray for you. Those people step up to support you, check in on you, and serve you. Friends inspire and motivate you.

You may not feel like eating healthy foods today, but if the friend you are meeting for lunch orders a healthy entrée, it will boost your decision to order the same. You may not feel like meditating on God's Word, but if you're going to church or a small group tonight, they will bring you into God's presence. The sense of community is why fitness classes and activity groups are so popular — they provide motivation for long-lasting change.

A safe group of friends is also a place where God promises to be with you. Jesus Christ made an incredible promise about it: "For where two or three gather together as my followers, I am there among them" (Matthew 18:20 NLT).

A team of friends will keep you on track for the race that God has given you to run. And you will do the same for others. This is the secret of The Daniel Plan — include friends with every other Essential, and you will see just how far you can go. Let's get healthy together.

## Reflect and Take a Step ...

Now it's time to assess where you are. Everyone has a different starting point, so make this very personal. How is your overall health? What changes do you want to start with? Using The Daniel Plan website, journal, or app, make some notes on where you are with each of the five Essentials you have just read about. Then, over the next forty days, keep tabs on how your choices and changes begin to restore your body and mind.

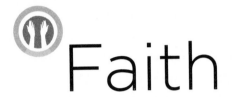

# Chapter 3

# Faith

*I can do all this through him who gives me strength (Philippians 4:13).*

Before you can make any healthy changes in your life, you must first believe those changes are possible.

Even more important, if you want God's help, you must trust him to give you his power to change. Jesus said, "According to your faith let it be done to you" (Matthew 9:29).

We call this the Faith Essential, and it is one of the key differences between The Daniel Plan and other approaches to better health. If you don't trust God to help you get healthy, all you are left with is willpower — and you know from experience that willpower doesn't usually last very long. You get tired of doing what's right, and you give up.

The Bible says, "Let's not get tired of doing what is good. At just the right time we will reap a harvest of blessing if we don't give up" (Galatians 6:9 NLT). But where do you get the power to keep on going? You get it from God, by asking him to empower you and trusting in him moment by moment.

God can make changes in your life that you have never dared to even dream of. He specializes in miracle makeovers. "God can do anything, you know — far more than you could ever imagine or guess or request in your wildest dreams!" (Ephesians 3:20 MSG). That is a power that you cannot find anywhere else.

Every year hundreds of self-help books are published. Many of them offer excellent advice, but most of them lack the most important ingredient: explaining where you get the power to change. They tell you what to do, but do not provide the power to do it. That can be frustrating.

For instance, have you ever tried to give up caffeine or sugar? You may succeed for a few days or a few weeks, but then stress hits, and you wind up needing a pick-me-up. Before you know it, you have been drinking two double lattes a day for a week straight. Or have you ever tried to forgive someone who has never admitted his wrong against you? You put your mind to it and feel at peace for a short time. Then something triggers your memory, the hurt and anger return, and you think, *I will never be able to forgive that person.* You're right. You can't do it without God's help.

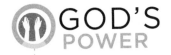

# GOD'S POWER

**PROVERBS 16:9 SAYS,** "We plan the way we want to live, but only God makes us able to live it" (MSG). The reason we eventually fail at all our good resolutions is because we don't depend on God. How many times have you started off a new year with a new resolution or a new desire or a new diet, and only a few weeks later you're right back in the same spot? You need willpower, but you also need more than that for a lifetime change. God says, "Don't depend on your own power or strength, but on my Spirit" (Zechariah 4:6 CEV).

Think about this: What positive changes in your life could happen if you relied on God's unlimited power instead of your limited willpower. The Faith Essential in The Daniel Plan means that you won't be doing it on your own. God will help you as you rely on him and trust him to give you the ability and power to change what you want to change. I explain this in detail in *The Purpose Driven Life*:

> Jesus said, "With man this is impossible, but with God all things are possible" (Matthew 19:26).

> Only the Holy Spirit has the power to make the changes God wants to make in our lives.... We allow Christ to live *through* us ... through the choices we make. We choose to do the right thing in situations and then trust God's Spirit to give us his power, love, faith, and wisdom to do it. Since God's Spirit lives inside of us, these things are always available for the asking.[1]

God understands you better than you understand yourself. God knows what makes you tick — he knows what energizes you, what fatigues you, what makes you sick, and what makes you operate at your best. Doesn't it make sense to trust him to help you?

God has been there every moment of your life. He watched you being formed in your mother's womb and watched you take your first breath. That means he cares about every detail, including your health. So why would you attempt to get healthy — something God clearly desires for you — without relying on him?

The fact is, you will never reach your optimum health without paying attention to the spiritual dimensions of your life. You have a body, but you are far more than just a body. Every area of your life affects every other area. For instance, it's hard to be spiritually strong and mentally alert when you are emotionally stressed or physically fatigued. If you are spiritually and emotionally weak or ill, your body cannot perform at its peak. The Daniel Plan is about your total health, not just your physical fitness. For this reason, we must start with your relationship to God — the Creator who designed you, knows best how your body was made to operate, and has the power to help you make the changes that you want to see.

## YOU NEED GOD TO CHANGE

Without God's power in your life, you are just running on your own energy. God never meant for you to do that. It's like having a laptop that's unplugged; the battery will eventually drain and shut down the computer. Why would you live like that when God created you for so much more?

If you find yourself tired all the time, one reason may be that you are trying to solve all your problems, fulfill your responsibilities, and make all your changes on your own. One clue that this may be happening is when you worry more than you pray.

Think of it this way: You have a small battery inside you. It has a limited amount of energy. When it depletes, you shut down. At the same time, God offers you access to his unlimited power plant. All you need to do is plug in — and the power cord is prayer.

Stop trying, and start trusting. The key to a faith-filled life is not in trying harder. It's not in psyching yourself up, but in relaxing in God's grace, so he can do through you what he desires to do. Philippians 2:12 – 13 says, "Be energetic in your life of salvation, reverent

## God Got Me off the Couch

"The weekend that Pastor Rick spoke about the need to be healthy to fulfill God's plan for our lives, he challenged those of us who were carrying a few extra pounds to write down the number of pounds we wanted to lose by Christmas and drop a card in the basket. I wrote down '25 pounds,' hopeful that this would finally be the time it worked. At age 36, I was 288 pounds, probably headed toward all the health problems that overweight people have.

"I had no idea about the journey God was going to take me on. I didn't feel any different. I didn't hear God speak to me. I just dropped a card in a basket. God knew what I did. God had just enrolled me in what I like to call Daniel Plan 1.0. When I woke up the next morning, God had taken over my physical life. I had not exercised in years. That day, I started small by going for a walk. I had not eaten well — ever. That day, I began to view food differently. My lifelong battle with my weight changed that day because God grabbed hold of me and changed my heart. As I write this note, I am 70 pounds lighter than I was six years ago.

"God got me off the couch six years ago, and He will get the credit when I cross the finish line of Ironman Arizona. I have swum, biked, and run nearly 20,000 miles in the last six years. Along the way, I have said many prayers of thanks that God has given me the ability and desire to be fit. I know of no greater way to worship God than to be outside enjoying His creation doing what He created me to do."

— Joel Guerra

and sensitive before God. That energy is God's energy, an energy deep within you" (MSG).

Later, in the same book, Paul says this: "I have the strength to face all conditions by the power that Christ gives me" (Philippians 4:13 GNT). Notice that it doesn't say, "I have the strength for *most* conditions." It says *all* conditions. That includes breaking bad habits and creating healthy ones.

Living by faith means you are attempting to do something you cannot do yourself. Anything you can do by your own effort obviously doesn't require faith. But in the areas of your life that seem unchangeable — the intractable problems, the persistent areas of failure, the stubborn bad habits that won't respond to willpower — these things require a power greater than you possess. Just ask anyone who has overcome an addiction through the Celebrate Recovery program.

You may have had so many failures at changing the way you eat or exercise or think or act that the possibility of lasting change feels like an unreachable goal. Well, to be honest with you, it probably will be — unless you plug into God's power. What is impossible from a human standpoint is easy to God. With God, today's impossibility is tomorrow's miracle. Are you ready for one?

The Bible says, "Without faith it is impossible to please God" (Hebrews 11:6). It will take faith to achieve and maintain the total health that God desires for you. But it begins with admitting that you don't have enough power on your own to become all you're meant to be. People of faith are those who admit that they can't do it on their own. The journey starts with humility. Have you taken that first step yet?

For some people, it takes years of frustration and failures before they can admit that willpower alone doesn't work to make the deepest changes. We need both a savior and a manager (or "Lord") of our lives. Fortunately, God came to earth in Jesus to fulfill that role for us. It's the reason Christmas is the biggest holiday on the planet. If we didn't need a savior, God would not have wasted the time and energy to send one 2,000 years ago.

## THE LOVE BEHIND THE POWER

To really understand God's power, you have to know and believe his love for you. God loves you so much that he freely gives his power to work in your life. God proved his love by sending Jesus to die on the cross *for you*, even before you knew how much you needed that to be done for you. How great is God's love for you?

Ephesians 3:17 – 19 says, "Then Christ will make his home in your hearts as you trust in him. Your roots will grow down into God's love and keep you strong. And may you have the power to understand, as all God's people should, how wide, how long, how high, and how deep his love is. May you experience the love of Christ, though it is too great to understand fully" (NLT). This verse reveals that God's love for us is far greater than our human brains can comprehend. It is four-dimensional:

**God's love is wide enough to be everywhere.** There is no place on this planet where God's love isn't present. There is no place in the universe where God's love ends. In your life, you will go through many experiences that leave you feeling sad, discouraged, or alone. But you're not alone. There will never be a moment in your life when God is not paying attention to you.

### Faith Power

Kalei Kekuna had always struggled with her body image and being self-conscious. For many years she battled with an eating disorder. As she realized God's power and love through The Daniel Plan, her focus shifted. "I learned that God loves me exactly the way that I am, unconditionally. It's not necessarily about losing weight or looking a certain way. It's more about making healthy choices that help me follow God's plan for me.

"I wake up every morning and say, 'God, I need help with this. Can you please just be there with me through this day as I make healthy choices and as I choose to go to the gym versus sitting on my couch, and as I choose the healthy salad versus the donut?' Just knowing that he's there the entire time helping me through this was a huge change for me."

**God's love is long enough to last forever.** Human love often withers and dies, because it is conditional. People say, "I love you if . . ." or "I love you because . . . ," and when circumstances change, the love evaporates. But God's love is unconditional, so he will never, never stop loving you. You cannot make God stop loving you, because his love is based on who he is, not what you do. It is based on his character, not your conduct. This doesn't mean that God approves or likes everything you do. He doesn't. But your sin does not stop him from loving you. It is this unconditional grace of God, not conditional approval, that is the foundation of The Daniel Plan.

**God's love is deep enough to handle anything.** No matter what hurt you have experienced in the past, what problems you're going through right now, or what pain you will face in the future, you can count on God's love. There may be days when you feel you have hit bottom and could not possibly go any lower. Well, beneath what feels like the bottom is the bedrock of God's love. Nothing is deeper than his love for you.

**God's love is high enough to overlook my sins.** Jesus said, "I did not come to judge the world, but to save the world" (John 12:47). Have you accepted his forgiveness and salvation by faith? This is where the Faith Essential begins. You can't have the power of God in your life without Jesus in your life. It all starts with a relationship. Not rules. Not regulations. Not rituals. Not religion. It's all about a relationship to God through his Son, Jesus.

God's laws and commandments simply show our inability to do what's right without his grace and power in us:

> Its purpose was to make obvious to everyone that we are, in ourselves, out of right relationship with God, and therefore to show us the futility of devising some religious system for getting by our own efforts what we can only get by waiting in faith for God to complete his promise. For if any kind of rule-keeping had power to create life in us, we would certainly have gotten it by this time! (Galatians 3:21 MSG).

Resolutions and rules aren't enough to change the human heart. For example, the government can create a law that makes racism illegal, but no law will transform a bigot into a kind, loving person. That kind of heart transformation requires the love of God inside.

The beginning of healthy change starts in the heart. If you haven't yet opened your heart to God's love, I urge you to do so right now, before you read another chapter. It's the healthiest choice you will ever make. When you invite Jesus to be the Savior and Lord (manager) of your life, your past is forgiven, you get a new purpose for living, and you get a home in heaven. In addition, you plug into God's power to change your life.

> The Bible promises, "You will know ... how very great is his power at work in us who believe. This power ... is the same as the mighty strength which he used when he raised Christ from death" (Ephesians 1:18 – 20 GNT).

Here is a prayer I would urge you to pray. The words are not as important as the attitude of your heart. If you're in a place where you can read this prayer aloud, I encourage you to do so. Otherwise, read it quietly to yourself:

Dear God, thank you for creating me and loving me so that I can have a relationship with you. Thank you for understanding the frustration I have felt in failing to change things in myself that need changing. I realize that without your help I am powerless to change my deepest habits, hurts, and hang-ups. I need a Savior, and I thank you for sending Jesus to die on the cross for me.

Jesus, I need your presence, your power, and your purpose in my life. I want to turn from my plans to your plan, and from depending on my power to your power. From now on, I want you to be the Lord and manager of my life. In faith, I humbly ask you to forgive my sins and my failures and help me to become what you intended for me to be. For the rest of my life, I want to get to know you better so I can trust you more. I pray this in your name. Amen.

## HOW GOD'S POWER WORKS

Philippians 2:12 – 13 explains that lasting change and spiritual growth come as a result of our cooperation with God. We cannot achieve that on our own, but he will not do it without our cooperation. God supplies the resources and power for change, but we must make choices to activate those things in our lives. To put it another way: "Continue to work out your salvation with fear and trembling, for it is God who works in you to will and to act in order to fulfill his good purpose."

Notice two phrases: *work out* and *work in*. We are commanded to *work out* while God *works in* us! That's the cooperation required for change. What does it mean to work out your salvation? Well, it doesn't mean "work FOR" your salvation, because salvation cannot be earned. "For it is by grace you have been saved, through faith — and this is not from yourselves, it is the gift of God — not by works, so that no one can boast" (Ephesians 2:8 – 9).

When you do a physical *workout*, you develop the muscles God has already given you. In these verses the Bible is talking about a spiritual workout — not to earn or gain your salvation, but to grow and develop the new life God has given you. So, in your growth and change, God has a part and you have a part. You work out, and God works in!

Let's first look at God's side of the equation (what he works in), then we will look at our side of the equation (what we work out).

**1. God uses his Word to change us.** The first tool God uses in changing us is the Bible. Through Scripture he teaches us how to live and how to change. Second Timothy 3:16 – 17 tells us, "All Scripture is inspired by God and is useful to teach us what is true and to make us realize what is wrong in our lives. It corrects us when we are wrong and teaches us to do what is right. God uses it to prepare and equip his people to do every good work" (NLT). Another way of saying this is that God's Word shows us (1) the path to walk on, (2) when we have gotten off the path, (3) how to get back on the path, and (4) how to stay on the right path.

If you are serious about changing your life in any significant way, you are going to have to get into the Bible. You need to read it, study it, memorize it, meditate on it, and apply it. Jesus said, "Then you will know the truth, and the truth will set you free" (John 8:32). Sometimes learning the truth about ourselves first makes us miserable — because we want to deny it — but ultimately, the truth is liberating.

The first element of The Daniel Plan is faith, and the way you grow your faith is by filling your mind with the truth of God's Word.

**2. God uses his Spirit to change us.** The second resource God uses to change us is his Spirit within us. He doesn't just offer advice from the sidelines. When we commit ourselves to Christ, the Holy Spirit comes into our lives to empower and direct us (Romans 8:9 – 11). The Spirit of God gives us his strength to do what is right. Second Corinthians 3:18 says,

> "Faith cometh by hearing, and hearing by the Word of God" (Romans 10:17 KJV).

"As the Spirit of the Lord works within us, we become more and more like him and reflect his glory even more" (NLT).

Note that God's goal in all the changes we make is that we become more and more like Christ. God's number one purpose in our lives is to make us like Jesus Christ. The Spirit of God uses the Word of God to make the child of God more like the Son of God. And what is Jesus like? His life on earth embodied the nine fruits of the Spirit listed in Galatians 5:23 – 24: love, joy, peace, patience, kindness, goodness, faithfulness, gentleness, and self-control.

**3. God uses circumstances to change us.** God's ideal way to change us is through the Bible so that we can find out how we should live and then through his indwelling Spirit, who enables us to do it. Unfortunately, we can be too often stubborn, and we don't change that easily or quickly. Bad habits get ingrained. So God brings in a third tool to work on us: circumstances! This refers to the problems and pressures, heartaches and hard times, difficulties and stress that we all experience.

Problems always get our attention, and the more painful they are, the more we pay attention. C. S. Lewis noted that God whispers to us in our pleasure but shouts to us in our pain. It often takes a painful situation to get our attention. We all know the truth of Proverbs 20:30: "Sometimes it takes a painful experience to make us change our ways" (GNT). The truth is, we are more likely to change because we feel the heat than because we see the light! People rarely change until the pain exceeds the fear of change.

The interesting thing about how God uses circumstances is that their source makes no difference at all to him. We often bring problems on ourselves by our own faulty decisions, poor choices, bad judgments, and sins. Other times our problems are caused by other people. Sometimes the devil causes things to happen to us as he did to a man named Job in the Bible. But God says the source of the circumstance is irrelevant. He will still use it for your good and your growth if you cooperate with him.

Romans 8:28 – 29 is one of the great promises of the Bible: "We know that God is always at work for the good of everyone who loves him. They are the ones God has chosen for his purpose, and he has always known who his chosen ones would be. He had decided to let them become like his own Son" (CEV).

### Shoe Lesson

"I wear shoes for comfort, not for style, and once they get broken in and very comfortable, I hate to give them up. A few years ago, I had a pair of shoes that I wore almost every day for over a year. They finally started getting holes in the bottom of them, but they were so comfortable that I continued to wear them. I just wouldn't cross my legs when sitting on a platform so the audience couldn't see the holes! I knew I needed to buy new shoes, but I kept putting it off. Then it rained for an entire week. After four days of soggy socks, I got motivated to buy some new shoes.

"The first step in change is usually discomfort!"

—Pastor Warren

God promises that he will fit everything — even your setbacks, relapses, and failures — into his plan and purpose for your life. God loves to turn stumbling blocks into stepping-stones and crucifixions into resurrections.

So God shows you how to change through the truth in the Bible, then his Spirit within you gives you the power to change. But if you ignore these, God will gladly use circumstances to get your attention. God loves you whatever way you are, but he loves you too much to let you stay that way, and he will use whatever it takes to help you grow to spiritual maturity.

# 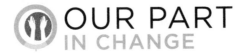OUR PART
## IN CHANGE

**IF GOD'S RESPONSIBILITY** is to provide life-changing truth, Holy Spirit power, and custom-made experiences to help you change and grow, then what is your responsibility for personal change? You must develop three spiritual habits that will deepen your faith and develop your spiritual strength.

## CHOOSE TO FILL YOUR MIND WITH GOD'S WORD EVERY DAY

Change is a matter of choice. We can't just passively sit around doing nothing and expect our lives to get better. We must make healthy choices to use the resources God gives us, and the first healthy choice is to carefully choose what we think about.

It is often said, "You're not what you think you are, but what you think about, you are!" Did you get that? If you are going to change your life, you must first change the way you think — your perceptions about God, about yourself, about life, about food, about health, and about everything else. Change always begins with new thinking. We must change the patterns of our mind. (We will look at this more in chapter 6 on Focus.)

The biblical word for personal change is *repentance*. Most people completely misunderstand the term. The popular conception of repentance is "Stop sinning! Quit doing bad things!" But the word actually means *to change your mind*. It comes from the Greek word *metanoia*, which means to change your perspective, think in a different way, make a mental U-turn.[2] Of course, if you change your mind, your behavior will follow, but repentance starts in the mind, not in actions.

Choosing to change your perspective and what you think about

### The Start of My Change

"When I repented and accepted God's gift of salvation by grace, I changed my perspective on a lot of things. I began to think differently about God, good and evil, my past, my present, my future, my relationships, my money, my time, sex, work, play, and everything else.

"When you truly repent, you see everything differently. Having a new perspective changes your values. As the apostle Paul said, 'I once thought all those things were so very important, but now I consider them worthless because of what Christ has done' (Philippians 3:7 NLT)."

— Pastor Warren

is your first responsibility in getting healthy. The Bible teaches that the way you think determines the way you feel, and the way you feel determines the way you act. If you want to change any behavior, you must start by challenging your unhealthy perspective on that subject. For example, if you have difficulty controlling your anger, don't start with your actions; instead, begin with identifying and changing the thoughts that prompt you to anger. Romans 12:2 says that we are transformed by the renewing of our mind. We are not transformed by an act of our will, but by repentance — seeing everything from God's perspective.

Imagine that you have a speedboat with an autopilot that is set to head east across a lake, and you suddenly decide that you want to go west, in the exact opposite direction. What would you do?

You would have two options: The hardest way would be to grab the steering wheel and physically force the boat to go in the opposite direction than it was programmed to go. By sheer willpower you could force the boat to make a 180-degree turn. As long as you held onto the steering wheel, the boat would head in the new direction. But the entire time, you would feel the tension in your arms and body because you were forcing the autopilot to go against its programmed nature. You would feel stressed and uptight, and eventually you would get tired and let go of the steering wheel. At that point, the boat's autopilot would immediately return to heading east.

The simpler and easier way to change the direction of the boat is to change the autopilot. Then it will naturally head in the direction you want it to go.

For a similar reason, this is why diets, quit-smoking plans, and other self-help efforts based on willpower eventually fail. The entire time you are forcing yourself to change, you are under tension because your old thought patterns are unconsciously telling you to keep doing what you've always done. We get tired of doing what feels "unnatural" and soon quit exercising, or start smoking again, or return to our bad habits and destructive ways of relating to others. We are victims of our own autopilots that we have programmed by repetition.

Your autopilot is the collection of thoughts and ideas in your mind that you believe to be true about yourself and what feels natural. Complete this sentence ten times, and you will have a good idea of what your mental autopilot is: "It's just like me to ..."

> What you think determines the way you feel.
> What you feel determines the way you act.

The good news is that God can change your mental autopilot far faster than you can. He specializes in giving you a new mind-set. That new mind-set will change the way you feel, which will change the way you act. I pointed out earlier that Jesus said the truth sets you free. When you begin to renew your mind with God's Word, and you replace old lies, false ideas, and misconceptions with the truth, it will set you free from the habits and hang-ups that limit your life. Your actions will naturally begin to align with your new attitudes.

This process only happens when we follow God's instructions. God's Word gives us life-changing truth, but we must read it, study it, memorize it, meditate on it, and then practice it. When I use the word *meditation*, I am talking about biblical meditation as described in the book of Psalms, in Joshua 1:8, and in many other passages of the Bible.

In many ways, biblical meditation is the exact opposite of eastern or New Age meditation, which is about emptying your mind and repeating a single word or mantra. In contrast, biblical meditation means taking a verse of the Bible, such as a promise or a command or a story, and seriously pondering its meaning. You think through the implications for and application of God's truth to your life. This is the kind of meditation that David referred to when he repeatedly said, "I meditate on your Word day and night" (see Psalm 1:2; 119:148, etc.).

God makes some amazing promises to those who take the time to seriously think about his Word. Psalm 1:1 – 3 says, "Blessed is the one … whose delight is in the law of the LORD [the Bible], and who meditates on his law day and night. That person is like a tree planted by streams of water, which yields its fruit in season and whose leaf does not wither — whatever they do prospers." What a promise! Would

## Seeing Things Differently

As a pastor, Tom Crick noticed a change in his spiritual life as he started The Daniel Plan. "If you're constantly in the Bible, reading and doing your devotion time, all of a sudden you start to see things there that are really speaking to what you're doing in the rest of your life." Biblical principles that he would read before now had practical application to his health. Each day it was as if the Scriptures were encouraging him to eat better and boosting his energy. Then he started noticing the same thing happening with others who were doing The Daniel Plan.

"Like me, I saw people start to see things in the Scriptures that they didn't see before. They could [read] a Scripture and say, 'This applies to me, and this is how I'm getting through those tough times when I have a craving. [I saw others] using God's Word to help them…. What a difference when you really start to figure out what Scripture means to your life."

you like to succeed at everything you do? God makes that promise to those who meditate on the Bible.

So how do you learn to meditate on God's Word as David did? It's not hard at all. You focus your attention on a single truth from the Bible and then continue to think about it throughout your day. If you look in a dictionary, you will find that a synonym for *meditation* is the word *rumination*. Rumination is what a cow does when it chews its cud. A cow eats some grass, chews it up, then swallows it. The grass soaks in the stomachs for a while, then the cow burps it up again — with renewed flavor! The cow chews on it a while more and finally swallows it again. That process is rumination. That cow is extracting every ounce of nourishment it can from that grass as it digests it.

In a similar way, biblical meditation is truth digestion. You aren't putting your mind in neutral, but the exact opposite. Biblical meditation means engaging your mind to probe and consider and analyze what God has said in his Word. You think about a Bible verse over and over and over to digest its meaning and application to your life.

Philippians 4:6 – 7 explains the benefits of meditating on Scripture instead of worrying: "Don't worry about anything; instead, pray about everything. Tell God what you need, and thank him for all he has done. Then you will experience God's peace, which exceeds anything we can understand. His peace will guard your hearts and minds as you live in Christ Jesus" (NLT).

### Easier Than You Think

You may be thinking that biblical meditation is a difficult skill to develop, but you actually already know how to do it if you know how to worry! When you take a fear or a problem or a negative thought and think about it over and over, that's called worry. When you take a verse of Scripture and think about it over and over, that's called biblical meditation.

If you are serious about improving your life and your health, you need to invest a minimum of 10 minutes a day reading the Bible, meditating on what you've read, writing down what you learn, and then talking to God in prayer about it. This healthy habit is called "daily quiet time." If you would like to learn more about how to set up and structure a daily quiet time, email me, PastorRick@saddleback.com, and I will gladly send you a booklet I wrote nearly forty years ago that has helped millions of people begin this habit. You can also use *The Daniel Plan Journal* to get started. You will be amazed at how much it transforms your life.

## CHOOSE TO DEPEND ON GOD'S SPIRIT EVERY MOMENT

Everyone who trusts Christ to save them receives his Holy Spirit in their lives, but few people experience the power of the Holy Spirit because they still depend on their own power instead. Learning to depend on God's Spirit to guide you, strengthen you, empower you, and use you is the second habit you must develop for spiritual strength.

Jesus gives a beautiful illustration of this in John 15. He compares our spiritual life to a grapevine and its branches. Jesus said, "I am the vine, and you are the branches. If you stay joined to me, and I stay joined to you, then you will produce lots of fruit. But you cannot do anything without me" (John 15:5 CEV).

No grape branch can produce fruit without staying connected to the main vine, and you cannot produce spiritual fruit while disconnected from God's Spirit. The fruitfulness of your life will depend on how dependent you are on the Holy Spirit. Attempting to bear fruit (and making positive changes) on your own power is as foolish as tying apples on the branches of a dead apple tree. From a distance, it might look as if the tree is alive and fruitful, but on closer inspection, people would realize the fruitfulness is fake.

Many "religious" people try to fake fruitfulness. They tie on all kinds of good activities — such as attending church services, helping the poor, and being polite and generous to others — but there really is no spiritual life or power inside them, because they are not connected to God. All their "spiritual" activities are just for show. When you get close to them, you can see that they don't have a personal relationship with Jesus.

So how do you develop a vibrant, life-giving relationship to God? The same way you develop any other relationship! It takes time, it takes talking, and it takes trust. To develop a friendship with God, you have to be in continual conversation with him, listening to him through his Word and talking with him in prayer. If you are not talking to God throughout your day, you certainly aren't depending on him. Prayer is far more than a once-a-day quiet time or a memorized blessing before each meal. God wants to have a running conversation with you!

What should you pray about? Everything! Here's a simple rule: If it's worth worrying about, then it is worth praying about. If you prayed as much as you worry, you would have a whole lot less to worry about.

## My Daily Conversation

"As I work through my day, I often find myself praying after each task, 'What's next, Lord?' And before I walk into any room for a meeting, I always say a silent prayer, asking God to give me wisdom for that meeting. Prayer is the key to staying connected to God, and staying connected is the key to God's power and effectiveness. I recently tweeted this: 'Much prayer — much power. Little prayer — little power. No prayer — no power.' If I am not quietly talking to God as I do my work, I am not depending on him at that moment. And if I don't talk to God about what I'm doing, it shows that I'm doing it on my own power."

— Pastor Warren

## CHOOSE TO TRUST GOD
## IN EVERY CIRCUMSTANCE

You cannot control everything that happens to you. In fact, most of what happens around you is completely out of your control. But you do have control over two important factors: You control your response, and you control how much you choose to trust God, regardless of your circumstances.

Viktor Frankl, a Jew, was sent to one of the Nazi death camps of World War II. In his powerful classic, *Man's Search for Meaning*, Frankl wrote that while he was a prisoner at Dachau, the guards stripped him of everything he had. They took his identity. They took his wife and family. They took his clothes. They even took his wedding ring. But, he said, there was one thing that no one could take from him: his freedom to choose his response and attitude. He wrote, "They offer sufficient proof that everything can be taken from a man but one thing: the last of the human freedoms — to choose one's attitude in a given set of circumstances, to choose one's own way."[3] No guards could take that away from Viktor Frankl. It was his choice.

None of us knows what will happen in the future, but we can control how we react and respond. We choose whether something will make us bitter or better. God gave us that freedom, and he is watching how we respond to events that don't go our way. What matters in life is not so much what happens *to* us, but what happens *in* us.

One of the most famous examples of that principle is the story of Joseph in the Old Testament. Joseph was betrayed by his jealous older brothers and sold into slavery. Years later, when they met again, the

Sometimes circumstances that look as if they are meant to destroy us end up being situations that develop us. That is why James 1:2–4 says, "When troubles come your way, consider it an opportunity for great joy. For you know that when your faith is tested, your endurance has a chance to grow. So let it grow, for when your endurance is fully developed, you will be perfect and complete, needing nothing" (NLT).

brothers feared retaliation, but Joseph said, "You intended to harm me, but God intended it for good" (Genesis 50:20). That is true for you too. Over your lifetime you will encounter people who intend to hurt you. But God's purpose for your life is greater than any problem you face, and he intends to use it for good, as Romans 8:28 promises. Anyone can bring good out of good, but God can bring good out of bad — if you will trust him in every circumstance.

Circumstances are the third tool God uses to change us, grow us, and make us more like Christ. Knowing this keeps us from becoming resentful or bitter. Romans 5:3 – 4 says, "We also have joy with our troubles, because we know that these troubles produce patience. And patience produces character, and character produces hope" (NCV).

This has been God's plan from the very beginning. When God decided to create human beings, he also decided to make us in his own image (Genesis 1:27). What does that mean? Not that we will become gods (we won't), but that we will become godly, having the same moral qualities of love, kindness, goodness, justice, and integrity that God has. He wants us to develop Christ-like character, which is more important than our appearance, our achievements, or our acquisitions in life.

The reason why your character is so important is that you are going to take it to heaven. You are not taking your career to heaven. You won't take your car or clothes or any of the material things you have collected on earth. But you are taking your character! So ultimately, it is the most important thing you can develop on earth. The five Essentials of The Daniel Plan — Faith, Food, Fitness, Friends, and Focus — will do far more than help you get healthier physically. They will help you deepen your faith and develop your character, which, in the long run, will matter even more than how you feel here and now. Christ-like character will reap eternal rewards that you will enjoy forever.

We want you to remember a very important truth: God is not waiting for you to get physically healthy or spiritually mature before he starts loving you or enjoying you. He loves you right now, and he will be cheering you on at every stage of your growth and development.

He is not waiting for you to cross the finish line first. He is smiling at you as you run the race.

You might be thinking, *But what if I happen to stumble or fall in the race?* God will still love you. Imagine this scene: If parents are watching their child run in a race at school and the child stumbles and falls, what do loving parents do? They cheer even more loudly. They don't criticize or belittle the child. They yell, "I know you can do it! Get up! I believe in you! Don't be discouraged! It's just a minor setback! Keep going! I know you can make it to the finish line!"

That is what God is saying to you right now. "I'm proud of you for trying, and I'm going to be helping you. I will supply the power you need if you will spend time with me reading my Word every day, if you will depend on my Spirit inside you every moment, and if you will trust me to use every circumstance in your life for your good and growth."

So this is your moment to grasp God's love and power. The moment you get a clearer view and stronger foundation of faith. The moment when God starts to change you from the inside out.

### Reflect and Take a Step . . .

Faith is the foundation of The Daniel Plan, and learning to rely on God's power is the key to lasting change. Don't be afraid to share everything with God. He is waiting to hear from you. Start with this simple prayer:

"Father, I want to do what I need to get healthy and glorify you. I know I can't do this on my own. I've tried and I've failed, and I'm nervous that I will fail again. I'm willing to do my part, Lord, and I'm going to faithfully trust that you are working to help me succeed. I'm learning that you want me to succeed more than I do. Help me see your hand in this quickly, and keep me encouraged as I work toward better health. Amen."

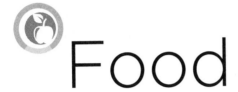

# Chapter 4

# Food

*So whether you eat or drink or whatever you do,
do it all for the glory of God (1 Corinthians 10:31).*

Most Americans are confused about food. Should you eat like a caveman and stick to meat, vegetables, and fruit and avoid all grains and dairy? Or eat only fruits, vegetables, and herbs like a gorilla? Low-carb or low-fat? What about food labels and calorie counts? What about all the health claims on the label? Or low-calorie or diet foods? What is the right diet?

Can we make sense of it all? It is not very easy, because the food and diet industry makes billions — in fact, more than $1 trillion — by keeping you guessing. It is good for them, but bad for you.

When you provide the conditions for a thriving human being and you remove the impediments to health, disease often simply goes away as a side effect. When you focus on health, healing and weight loss happen automatically. That is exactly what happens in The Daniel Plan.

The Daniel Plan was not designed as a weight-loss program. In fact, we never focused on weight, but on health. How do you create a healthy human? When we started the program at Saddleback Church, we designed it as a wellness program, combining the Essentials of faith, food, fitness, focus, and friends into a powerful potion of renewal and healing. Not only did the original participants lose more than 250,000 pounds in the first year, but they also reported improvement or resolution of chronic symptoms and diseases, including asthma, allergies, headaches, irritable bowel syndrome, acid reflux, autoimmune diseases, depression, heart disease, diabetes, hypertension, acne and skin issues such as eczema and psoriasis, brain fog, fatigue, and insomnia. They reported fuller engagement with their families, friends, church, and community, being better able to serve a higher purpose. Many lost well over 100 pounds and many type 2 diabetics got off insulin and multiple medications. We didn't have to treat all their diseases individually. Most chronic diseases and symptoms arise from the same common causes: imbalances in the five core Essentials.

Have you ever stopped to think about what food is, why we eat it, and what it does to us when we eat it? The link between food and our well-being is so immediate, so profound and direct, yet most of us have no idea that how we feel is linked to what we eat, that our various complaints and conditions and moods and energy (or lack of it) are driven by the fuel we put into our body.

Doctors rarely ask the simple question, "How do you create a healthy human?" Veterinarians study nutrition extensively. How do you get a horse to win the Kentucky Derby? You learn how to optimize its metabolism and health by the quality of the food you feed it.

> "Let food be thy medicine, and medicine be thy food."
> — Hippocrates, the ancient Greek physician

That is what we want for all of you — to optimize your health. We want you to love, enjoy, and celebrate food and use it to enrich and enliven you. Food can transform your health within a few weeks through the simple principles of The Daniel Plan.

The Daniel Plan is a way of life, or as some have called it, a *health-style* that takes the guessing out of eating and cooking. You can actually eat anything based on one rule: Eat real, whole food. Eat a colorful variety of real, whole foods from real ingredients that you can make yourself — or that are made by another human nearby.

If you want French fries, then make them yourself from whole potatoes and unrefined, unprocessed oil. Chances are you won't eat them every day, but you will enjoy them more and they will be much better for you.

Simple, real, fresh, delicious, nutrient-packed foods that are easy to cook, foods that come from a farmer's field rather than a factory, food that traveled the shortest distance from the field to your fork — that is what we should eat.

That's it — you can skip to the next chapter.

Well, maybe not yet. Unfortunately, most of us never learned what real food is, so just in case, we are going to lay it out for you in this chapter: What food is, what I should avoid, how I find the good stuff, and how I make my own meals.

# FOODS THAT HEAL:
## SO WHAT SHOULD WE EAT?

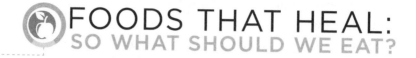

**WHAT IS FOOD? NOURISHMENT?** A source of energy or calories? A delightful pleasure?

Yes, it can be all of those things. But as a doctor who has dedicated his career to studying how food affects the body and contributes to or prevents disease, Dr. Hyman has a slightly different take on food: Food is medicine.

Food has the power to heal us. It is the most potent tool we have to help prevent and treat many of our chronic diseases — including diabetes and obesity. Truly, what you put on your fork dictates whether you are sick or well, slim or fat, depleted or energized.

How does food do all this? Through the groundbreaking science known as *nutrigenomics*. The molecules in your food do much more than provide fuel for your body. They provide instructions that tell every cell in your body what to do every moment. More than 95 percent of chronic illness is not related to your genes, but to what those genes are exposed to in your lifetime. We call that the *exposome*.

> Food is medicine. It is the most powerful tool we have to combat chronic disease.

The exposome is the sum of everything you eat, breathe, drink, think, and feel, plus the toxins in our environment and even the 100 trillion bacteria that live inside your gut. This is good news because it means that you have almost complete control over your health. And the most important thing you do every single day to interact with your genes is eat.

So the next time you put something on your fork, imagine what your genes might feel. Would they like that extra large soda or cheesy corn chips, or would they prefer some sweet blueberries or sautéed broccoli with garlic and olive oil?

We want to teach you how to treat your body with respect and kindness. We will teach you what foods to choose to nourish yourself and which ones to avoid. Most of all, we will show you how to create a nurturing, peaceful relationship with food and cooking that will automatically lead to weight loss, radiant health, and an overall sense of well-being.

> "Food is our common ground, a universal experience."
>
> — James Beard

The Scriptures teach us how to live and love fully. But somehow we skip over the parts that instruct us to honor the vessel of the Holy Spirit, our body. Being in a food coma from eating sugar and junk food, having your brain chemistry hijacked by hyper-processed, hyper-palatable, hyper-addictive foods prevents you from fully inhabiting your body and your mind. If the food you are eating is making you sick and unfocused and makes you so sluggish that if you happen to get the urge to exercise you instead lie down until it goes away, living a fully engaged and God-honoring life is difficult.

Real food has the power to give you your life back and more fully engage in the purpose for your life. The reason to do it is not to fit in your jeans or look good in a dress, but to be awake to the beauty and miracle of life, to be able to live with purpose, to love, serve, connect, and celebrate the gifts God has given you.

If you nourish your body with high-quality ingredients from real food, not only will you increase your energy, lose weight, and reverse many chronic illnesses, but you will also feel lighter and more motivated to exercise, your mood will lift, and your brain will have better clarity, allowing you to clear out the debris in the way of your relationships with others and God.

So what do we mean by "real" food? Anything that is whole, fresh, and unprocessed. Stuff that your great-grandmother would recognize

## Changing Control

"My biggest health achievement so far has been to lose over 150 pounds," Chloe Seals says. "I didn't know it at the time, but my doctor told me I was considered diabetic in 2010 when I weighed 277 pounds. Changing my eating habits and making healthier food choices has resulted in completely eliminating diabetes. I feel like I've gained my life back, and I feel more in control over what I eat instead of comfort and the lure of foods controlling me.

"I have learned to enjoy a variety of foods that I prepare for myself as well as my two kids. I feel better about myself instead of always feeling self-conscious. My greatest motivation comes from my kids and wanting to be healthy as long as I can so I can be there for them."

as food. A chicken, a vegetable, a bean, a nut, a grain, a fruit, an egg. Everything else is fake food that depletes energy and health. Real food heals. Real food nourishes.

The good news is that the list of real food is short, easy to understand, and easy to identify. Unfortunately, though, many of us are not well acquainted with real food. We have outsourced our cooking to the food industry for packaged, processed, and prepared convenience foods and to fast-food restaurants and convenience stores. But there is nothing convenient about feeling disconnected, sluggish, slothful, foggy, or depressed or having the diseases you get and medications you have to take when you fuel up with "convenient food."

Let's debunk one myth up front. We have been led to believe that eating well is expensive and that cooking your own food takes too much time. The facts are quite different. The research shows that you can eat well and in less time for less money than buying processed foods.[1] With a few simple tricks, you can shop well, cook simply, and eat better for less in the same time it takes to hit a fast-food drive-through window and eat your meal. More importantly, real food tastes better and is more nourishing and satisfying. It can even eliminate your cravings.

The Daniel Plan focuses on the core food groups of healthy carbs, healthy fats, healthy protein, healing spices, drinks, and super foods. And The Daniel Plan gives an easy guideline to use for any meal:

- 50 percent non-starchy veggies
- 25 percent healthy animal or vegetable proteins
- 25 percent healthy starch or whole grains
- Side of low-glycemic fruit
- Drink — water or herbal teas

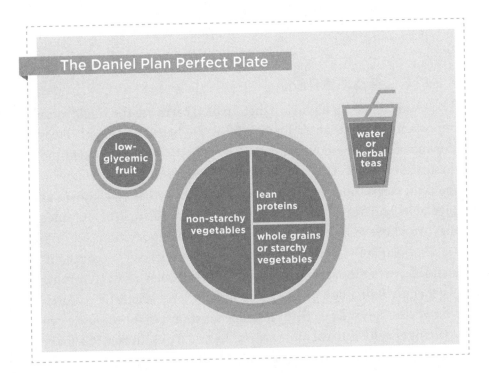

The Daniel Plan Perfect Plate

low-glycemic fruit

water or herbal teas

lean proteins

non-starchy vegetables

whole grains or starchy vegetables

## TOP 10 CHOICES IN EACH FOOD GROUP to Get You Started

| NON-STARCHY VEGGIES | PROTEIN | STARCH OR GRAIN | LOW-GLYCEMIC FRUIT |
| --- | --- | --- | --- |
| Asparagus | Beans | Beets | Apples |
| Bell peppers | Beef | Brown or black rice | Blackberries |
| Broccoli | Chicken | Carrots | Blueberries |
| Cauliflower | Eggs | Buckwheat | Gogi berries |
| Collard greens | Halibut | Green peas | Grapefruit |
| Cucumbers | Lentils | Corn | Plums |
| Green beans | Nuts | Quinoa | Kiwi |
| Kale | Salmon | Sweet potatoes | Nectarines |
| Spinach | Seeds | Turnips | Peaches |
| Zucchini | Turkey | Winter squash | Raspberries |

## THE GOOD CARBS

The Daniel Plan is a high-carb diet. In fact, carbs are the single most important food you can eat for long-term weight loss and health. Does this mean load up on cereal, bread, rice, pasta, cookies, cakes, and donuts? Sorry, no. All plant foods contain carbohydrates. You want the right carbs: unrefined, unprocessed carbs, otherwise known as vegetables and fruits. Whole grains and beans are also carbs, but since they are a little more starchy should be eaten in moderation.

Unfortunately, less than 10 percent of Americans eat the recommended five to nine servings of fruits and vegetables a day. (A serving is generally half a cup or one piece of fruit.) Yet scientific research overwhelmingly tells us that the single most important thing we can do for our health is to eat more vegetables and fruits. In fact, it is about the only thing that every nutritional philosophy agrees upon.

Plant foods contain a rich combination of blood-sugar-balancing, anti-inflammatory, detoxifying compounds called phytonutrients. Inflammation has been linked to most of the diseases of aging, including heart attacks, diabetes, cancer, and dementia. In fact, being overweight is a chronic inflammatory state. Vegetables and fruits contain nature's most powerful anti-inflammatories.

Plant foods are the main source of vitamins and minerals in your diet. These vitamins and minerals run every chemical reaction in your body; they are the grease that lubricates the wheels of your metabolism. The fiber in plant foods is necessary to keep your digestive system healthy, feed the good bacteria that keep inflammation down, and help balance blood sugar. Most Americans get 8 to 12 grams or less, while we really need 30 to 50 grams of fiber per day.

> "Then God said, 'I give you every seed-bearing plant on the face of the whole earth and every tree that has fruit with seed in it. They will be yours for food'" (Genesis 1:29).

The good news is that you get unlimited refills on vegetables. Think "binge on broccoli." (Okay, so broccoli may not sound that exciting, but stick with us!) When thinking about dinner, think about cooking two or three different kinds of vegetables or trying some raw varieties with a delicious dip, such as hummus or homemade salsa. (See chapter 10 for recipes.) When eating out, order two or three sides

## Boost Your Fiber

Add the following to your diet to increase your fiber:

- Whole grains such as quinoa or brown rice
- Vegetables, vegetables, vegetables
- Flax seeds (grind them and sprinkle on salads or fruit)
- Legumes — also known as beans and peas

of vegetables and skip the bread and pasta, which are proven to pack on the pounds and cause diabetes.

In fact, these plant foods should make up 50 percent of your diet. It's a big change for most people, but the closer you can come to upsizing the veggies and complementing with fruits, the more you will improve your health (and the health of the planet to boot).

When you get used to real foods, then we encourage you to focus on one simple principle: Focus on foods that don't raise your blood sugar or don't raise it quickly. This concept is called the Glycemic Index or glycemic load of foods. For example, white bread is a carb that raises your blood sugar more and faster than even table sugar, while crunchy green veggies barely make a dent in your sugar levels. Both are carbs, but act very differently calorie for calorie.

## THE GLYCEMIC INDEX

The Glycemic Index (GI) is a nutritional tool to identify how carbohydrates affect our blood sugar levels. Carbs with a low GI (55 or less) don't make our blood sugar levels rise too high, but provide sustained energy. Carbohydrates with a high GI (70 or more) cause our blood sugar levels to rise higher for a longer period. One of the best strategies for keeping blood sugar low is to incorporate low GI foods into your daily eating plan. These are some of the health benefits:

- Helping you avoid getting into a food emergency because you feel satisfied
- Keeping your insulin levels low, which helps burn fat easier
- Helping you to release body fat and keep lean muscle tissue
- Reducing your triglycerides, total and bad (LDL) cholesterol
- Increasing your levels of good (HDL) cholesterol
- Lessening your risk of developing type 2 diabetes
- Limiting your risk of developing cardiovascular disease
- Sustaining your energy levels longer, ultimately enhancing your mental and physical performance

## Top 10 Tips for Low-Glycemic Eating

1. Follow The Daniel Plan plate.
2. Fill half your plate with colorful vegetables.
3. Limit starchy vegetables such as potatoes, winter squash, or cooked beets (only ¼ of your plate).
4. Limit (or eliminate) sugar and flour products.
5. Eat protein for breakfast such as a whole food protein shake (see page 317 for a recipe), whole eggs, or an omelet, or have dinner for breakfast. Or incorporate more nuts and seeds into breakfast.
6. Add good fats to your diet such as extra-virgin olive oil, avocados, nuts and seeds, and extra-virgin coconut butter.
7. Replace starchy pasta choices with some gluten-free grains such as buckwheat, black or brown rice, or quinoa.
8. Eat beans such as lentils or chickpeas.
9. Choose a lean protein source (animal or plant) at every meal.
10. Carry snacks such as nuts and veggies with hummus to avoid a food emergency.

Breakfast Swap: Choose a whole grain breakfast, such as steel-cut oats with almonds and berries, instead of your favorite boxed cereal.

## THE CALORIE MYTH

Now is the time for us to blow up the calorie myth. Here's the myth: All calories are created equal.

The lesson we have all learned is that calories are a form of energy, and according to the laws of physics, a calorie is a calorie — the amount of energy required to raise the temperature of one liter of water by one degree centigrade. This law is true for physics, but all bets are off when you put biology in the mix. If it was all about "eat less, exercise more," we would all do it and be skinny and fit. But there are different kinds of calories: healing calories and disease-causing calories. Let us explain.

Let's compare a 20-ounce soda with 240 calories to the equivalent number of calories from broccoli (which is about 7.5 cups). The soda has no fiber and no vitamins or minerals, but has 15 teaspoons of sugar in the form of high fructose corn syrup, caffeine, and phosphoric acid — which causes osteoporosis. The sugar in the soda spikes your insulin, causes a fatty liver, increases triglycerides, lowers good cholesterol, raises bad cholesterol, increases cortisol (the stress hormone), and causes diabetes, heart disease, cancer, and dementia.

The broccoli (if you could actually eat the 7.5 cups!) has the same number of calories but about ½ teaspoon natural sugar and 35 grams fiber and is rich in vitamins and minerals, including folate and magnesium. Broccoli also contains powerful phytonutrients, which are healing plant compounds that help reduce your risk of cancer and boost your detoxification capacity. And broccoli has very little ability to raise your blood sugar. In fact, when it enters your body, the broccoli has the exact opposite effect of the soda. It creates health rather than destroys it. Same calories — very different results.

Clearly, all calories are not the same. It is a matter of quality. So we want to help you focus on becoming a "qualitarian."

## LOW-GLYCEMIC VEGETABLES

Low-glycemic vegetables are your new best friends. Go ahead and fill up on these life-giving plants. They should make up 50 percent of your plate. Keep a list of these as you walk through your grocery store, which is your new FARMacy, where you will find the best medicine for body and soul. Have two or three veggie dishes at dinner. Make a salad with arugula, artichokes, and avocados, and have a side of sautéed zucchini with garlic and olive oil and some roasted mushrooms. Go crazy!

Try some unusual and rare vegetables; they have much higher levels of nutrients and healing phytochemicals than the most common domesticated varieties.

Choose heirloom varieties when possible. Heirloom vegetables are unique varieties that predate all the major plant breeding of the last hundred years. For example: Cherokee purple tomatoes, Touchon carrots, or Black-seeded Simpson lettuce. They pack a more nutrient dense punch. You can often find them at farmer's markets or community-supported agriculture (CSA) programs.

## Mushrooms

Most of us are familiar with white button mushrooms and often use them raw in salads. Don't do that. They contain cancer-causing toxins when eaten raw. But there are other wonderful members of the mushroom family that have powerful anti-inflammatory, cancer preventing, and immune boosting properties. They are also full of minerals and are the best (and one of the only) vegetable sources of vitamin D. Try different and unique mushrooms. They have wonderful textures and flavors. Dr. Hyman puts them in a pan, drizzles with olive oil, garlic, and salt, and roasts them. They are amazing!

Try these mushrooms: oyster, porcini, shitake, maitake, and enoki. You can get these from Asian grocers and in many supermarkets today.

The one type of vegetable you can never get enough of is the cruciferous vegetable family, which includes kale, collards, broccolini, cabbage, Brussels sprouts, cauliflower, and bok choy. They contain powerful detoxifying chemicals called glucosinolates that prevent cancer and support your health. We recommend a cup or two every day.

### Sea Vegetables

Before you think this is too weird, you have probably already tried seaweed in sushi rolls. It's that black wrapping around the rice. Seaweed is one of the most nutrient dense, mineral rich, anti-cancer foods on the planet. If you have never tried sea vegetables, be adventurous. Try Seasnax, yummy, crunchy flavored nori snacks. You can add seaweeds such as kombu, arame, and wakame to soups and stews.

Look for them in the international or ethnic foods aisle of the grocery store; for more varieties check an Asian grocery or health food store. Adding kombu when you cook beans reduces their gas-producing effects.

## STARCHY VEGGIES

Most of us grew up on peas, carrots, and sweet corn as our side vegetables. These starchy plant foods have a place in a healthy diet. You still want to think of them as a side dish. They are sweeter, and for some people, they can raise blood sugar. But they are full of antioxidants and healing phytonutrients. Use starchy veggies — including beets, carrots, corn, green peas, Jerusalem artichokes/sun chokes, parsnips, potatoes, pumpkin, rutabagas, sweet potatoes or yams, turnips, winter squash — in a larger proportion to grains on your plate.

## PHYTONUTRIENTS

Now let's go back to phytonutrients. Your body is lazy — biochemically, that is. It doesn't do things one way that it can get done by some other means. The magic of your body is that you can use the power of plants to run important functions that keep you healthy. There is an entire class of compounds (phytonutrients) in our plant foods that work hard to reduce inflammation; rid our bodies of toxins; improve the way our bodies metabolize food and boost calorie burning;

optimize immune function; prevent cancer, heart disease, diabetes, and dementia; and contain powerful antioxidants that literally prevent our bodies from rusting and aging too fast.

*Detoxifying foods:* Cruciferous vegetables are the super detoxification foods. Other natural detoxifiers are green tea, watercress, dandelion greens, cilantro, artichokes, garlic, citrus peels, pomegranate, and even unsweetened cocoa powder (not the sugary hot chocolate kind).

For anti-inflammatory foods, think dark berries and cherries. Eat dark green leafy vegetables and orange sweet potatoes to cut down on inflammation. Curcumin is found in the yellow spice called turmeric and is used in curries and mustards. It is nature's ibuprofen and the most powerful anti-inflammatory. Add it to stir fries or when you cook grains or make curries.

### The Rainbow of Food

Eat from the rainbow of colors (and no, we don't mean Skittles) in the plant world, and you will be covering all the phytonutrient bases. Think reds, orange, yellows, greens, purple, blue — the darker and deeper the colors, the better they are for you.

Eat at least five to nine servings a day from the rainbow. Explore your supermarket and farmer's market to find unique and rare or heirloom vegetables. They pack more phytonutrient power in every bite.

*Antioxidant-rich foods:* These foods prevent aging and promote overall health. They are found in dark berries, black rice, beets, and pomegranates; orange and yellow vegetables such as winter squash; dark green leafy vegetables such as kale, collards, and spinach; and resveratrol-containing fruits such as purple grapes, blueberries, cranberries, and cherries.

*Hormone-balancing foods:* Foods such as miso, tempeh, and tofu (all of which are *whole* soy foods) and ground flax seeds help balance hormones and prevent cancer.

Many foods high in phytonutrients are also considered super foods. These are foods richest in high-quality protein, good fats, vitamins, and minerals. These are among the most health-promoting of all the foods you can eat. Visit The Daniel Plan website (*danielplan .com*) for a list of super foods.

## GRAINS

Whole grains can be part of a healthy diet, but in moderation. For some, grains can trigger spikes in blood sugar. The key is the amount

### Give Us Our Daily Bread

Jesus taught his disciples to pray, "Give us this day our daily bread." Eating bread is almost a religious commandment. Unfortunately, the bread we eat today is not the bread of biblical grains. Most bread now is highly processed and made from a different genetic strain of wheat that is higher in starch and contains gluten, a known inflammatory agent. (We will cover this more on page 122.)

Have you ever found yourself overeating from the bread basket? Processed or refined grains have all the fiber and nutrients stripped out of them, so they act just like sugar in your body. If something is made from flour (whether with gluten or gluten free), start thinking of it as a super sugar. If you want to lose weight or have known inflammatory health problems, it is best to eliminate it for a while or keep your intake to a minimum.

Here are a few tips to enjoy better quality bread:

- If you are not gluten sensitive (see page 119), then the best bread is whole kernel German rye bread (also

and what you eat them with. The ideal serving size for grains is ½ cup for men and ⅓ cup for women. You may tolerate more if you are a marathon runner, but for the average Joe or Joanna, the extra sugar can trigger insulin, weight gain, and inflammation.

The key is to eat only *whole* grains, not processed in any way. That means you buy them in their original form, such as oats, wheat berries, and even popcorn. Many packaged foods say "whole grains," but it is often a little whole grain flour mixed into white flour, sugary cereals, or other products. The ingredient list will tell you what's really in there.

If you have diabetes or pre-diabetes, you may not even be able to tolerate significant amounts of whole grains in your diet until you

made with flax and spelt), made from whole kernel grain, not whole grain flour. It is great toasted with anything on top.

- If you want regular flour bread, be sure that it contains no white flour (also labeled as "wheat flour") and is made from coarse whole grain flour, with extra protein and fiber ingredients such as nuts and seeds.

- Try sprouted whole grain breads such as Ezekiel 4:9 Whole Grain Sprouted Flax bread by Food for Life, if you are already healthy and fit.

- Change the way you think of bread. Think of it as a treat, to be used sparingly, ideally no more than one slice a day.

- Minimize flour-containing foods such as waffles, muffins, donuts, pretzels, and crackers.

- Try some of the non-flour crackers made from seeds and nuts.

correct the underlying metabolic imbalances. So the best grains are the gluten-free grains. Try low-glycemic grains such as black rice (also known as the emperor's rice), brown rice, red rice, buckwheat, and quinoa. Pastas cooked al dente (cooked just enough to retain some firm texture) are lower glycemic, but flour products should be considered a special treat that you only eat occasionally.

## FRUIT

Fruit is a wonderful source of powerful anti-inflammatory, antioxidant phytonutrient compounds. The darker and richer the colors, the more unique and wonderful the fruits, the more power-packed nutrition they contain. We focus on the lower sugar fruits such as berries and apples and pears and use the others as treats in smaller quantities. The average serving size is ½ cup or one piece of fruit. (If you are overweight or have blood sugar issues, then you want to be careful with fruit intake and limit it to one serving a day.) There are plenty of low-glycemic fruits.

- *Dark berries.* Blueberries, blackberries, and raspberries are rich in phytonutrients. You can get frozen organic versions and put them in shakes or even make great frozen desserts by putting them in the blender.

- *Stone fruit.* Plums, peaches, nectarines, cherries, and their variants are known as "stone fruit." They are healthy and full of fiber and healing chemicals and not too high in sugar.

- *Pomegranates, kiwis, papayas, and mangos* are also wonderful healing fruits.

- *Citrus fruits* such as grapefruit, oranges, lemons, and limes are great, but it's best to stay away from juices. They often have as much sugar as soda. (We will explain why when we talk about sugars.)

Limit high-sugar fruits. Melons, pineapple, and grapes are wholesome, but it's best to eat them in small quantities because of their high glycemic index. Also, dried fruit such as apricots, raisins, and currants are the highest in sugar, so use them sparingly. Many dried fruits also contain added sugar. Have one or two figs or dates or 2 tablespoons of raisins or currants as a treat, or mix a small amount with nuts and seeds to make your own trail mix.

## POWER UP WITH PROTEIN

The secret to optimal health, fewer cravings, balanced blood sugar, and losing weight is getting high-quality protein in every meal. But where should you get your protein? Americans have come to equate protein with beef, pork, or chicken, and meat is still the centerpiece of most dinner plates at home and in restaurants. The whole debate over veganism or paleo diets confuses people even more.

Science on both sides backs up the health claims. Some studies show that too much animal protein and dairy can cause heart disease and cancer. However, if you compare Spam or deli meats or even feed-lot factory-farmed beef to wild and lean buffalo/bison, grass-fed beef, or cage-free chicken, the effects are quite different.

The ironic thing is that vegan and paleo diets are closer to each other than the standard American diet full of sugar, trans fats, and processed foods. Vegan and paleo diets both emphasize whole foods, with lots of fruits and veggies, nuts, and seeds. Some people thrive on vegan diets, and some do poorly. Some feel weighed down by meat. We are all biochemically, metabolically, and genetically quite different.

Each of us has to listen to our own body and honor its uniquenesses. The body never makes a mistake. When we mindlessly put food in our mouths without considering if it is offering our body nutrition or healing, we compound our health issues. So we have to learn what our bodies thrive on and buy the best quality of it.

*Bottom line:* You want to include good quality protein with every meal, and it should make up about 25 percent of your plate or meal. A serving size is 4 to 6 ounces or about the size of your palm.

What follows are the best sources of protein in your diet.

## 1. HEALTHY ANIMAL PRODUCTS

If you enjoy animal proteins, whenever possible you want to choose the animal products that have the most to contribute to your health (and the least impact on the planet). You can't always find the cleanest or lowest impact, most humanely raised animal protein sources, but following these guidelines will shift the food production system, improve your health, and reduce negative environmental impact.

*Pick the right poultry.* Choose organic, grass-fed, free-range, and hormone-, antibiotic-, and pesticide-free poultry whenever you can. Chicken and turkey are good inexpensive sources of protein. A roast chicken dinner is cheaper than a trip to a fast-food joint for a family of four. Buy higher quality poultry; it should be available at your mainstream grocers. Why not even try ground turkey for your burgers once in a while? For turkey burger recipes, go to *danielplan.com* or *The Daniel Plan Cookbook*.

*Enjoy omega 3 eggs or free-range eggs.* Eggs were given a bad rap for a long time. Omega 3 eggs contain DHA, the ultimate omega 3 fat and brain food. Eggs *do not* raise your cholesterol; they do just the opposite. Egg yolks also contain choline and B vitamins. Stick with whole eggs, not egg whites.

*Go fish.* Fish is one of the best sources of protein and omega 3 fats. However, because of the contamination of our oceans and farmed

### Safe Fish and Meats

Download the app or reference card from *seafoodwatch.org*, or visit *cleanfish.com* to find fish companies and types of fish that are sustainably farmed and harvested (not overfished) and low in toxins.

See the Environmental Working Group's Meat Eater's Guide at *ewg.org/meateatersguide* to help you pick the best meat sources for you and the planet.

fisheries, finding safe fish is not as easy as it used to be. The best fish to eat are wild-caught and smaller, toxin-free fish such as sardines, tilapia, crawfish, and freshwater trout. Think small fish. If the whole fish can fit in your frying pan, it is probably safe to eat. It is best to stay away from fish with high mercury levels. For a handy wallet card listing fish with the lowest mercury content, go to *nrdc.org/health/effects/mercury/walletcard.PDF*.

*Get shelled.* Shrimp and scallops are also healthy forms of seafood low in toxins and high in good quality protein and minerals. Oysters are among the highest sources of zinc.

*Downsize your meat.* Choose quality over quantity. Small amounts of lean, organic, grass-fed, and hormone- and antibiotic-free lamb or beef can be a part of a healthy diet. You can even think about buying and freezing a whole animal with your extended family, friends, or church group. Consider trying leaner, more sustainably raised or wild animal products such as bison or buffalo or venison. Eat red meat no more than once or twice a week and no more than 4 to 6 ounces per serving. There are good sources at local health food stores, and many grocery stores are starting to carry better options.

Pork is the least healthy meat. Excess meat consumption has been associated with cancer, heart disease, and diabetes. Avoid charred or blackened meat, which causes cancer because overgrilling creates carcinogens.

## 2. VEGETARIAN SOURCES OF PROTEIN

*Go nuts.* Nuts can be part of your protein intake. They are a wonderful source of protein, fiber, minerals, and good fats that satisfy your appetite and reduce the risk of diabetes and heart disease. Nut butters are a great snack. Keep bulk nuts tightly sealed in the pantry or fridge. Eat walnuts, almonds, pecans, and macadamia nuts. Watch portion sizes. A serving is a handful or about 10–12 nuts. Buy raw or lightly toasted, unsalted nuts. Avoid nuts fried or cooked in oils.

*Seed your health.* Seeds are easy to add to salads, bean or grain dishes, and smoothies, or just enjoy a handful. Try pumpkin, sunflower, and sesame seeds, or add unusual seeds to your diet such as black sesame seeds. (Sprinkle them on eggs or into a stir fry.) Experiment with hemp, chia, and flax seeds; they are rich in omega 3 fats, minerals, and fiber.

*Enjoy soy.* This is a controversial topic, and many are worried about the harmful effects of soybeans on our health. But the science is straightforward. Stick with traditional whole soy products. These include tempeh, tofu, miso, and natto. They are broken down or fermented to make them easily digestible. Modern industrial soy products, extracted from soybeans in the process of creating soybean oil (which is then used to make trans fats), cause cancer and should be avoided. More than 90 percent of soy in the typical American diet is hidden and made from genetically modified or industrially refined soybeans. So avoid processed soy products, such as those found in deli-meat replacements, soy cheese, or meal-replacement bars.

### Beans

Baked beans full of sugar being served as a side to a processed hot dog is how most of us first "tasted" beans. But beans are a wonderful, inexpensive, power-packed source of protein, fiber, vitamins, and minerals. They don't spike blood sugar for most people, and some simple strategies can make them easier to digest. Buy canned precooked beans (preferably in BPA-free cans), or buy them in bulk and cook them yourself. If you cook them, add a piece of kombu (a seaweed), fennel seeds, or fresh ginger slices to the pot while the beans boil to improve digestibility. You can also take digestive enzymes to help your body digest the beans.

Try different varieties, such as chickpeas, adzuki, Anasazi, mung, kidney, black, or pinto beans, in soups, stews, and in salads. Lentils cook quickly and come in many varieties, including French, red, and regular.

*Bulk up on beans or legumes.* You can prepare these with a little planning by soaking them overnight and cooking in batches. This is the cheapest bang for your buck. Or you can buy canned beans in toxin-free (bisphenol A-free, or BPA-free) cans for a quick meal or addition to salads, soups, or stews.

## HEALING FATS

On The Daniel Plan you get to enjoy many healthful fats. We used to think that fat is all bad and causes heart disease. Here's the skinny on fats. The good fats such as omega 3s from fish, nuts, seeds, avocados, olives and extra-virgin olive oil, and coconut butter (a plant-derived saturated fat) have been proven to reduce diabetes, heart disease, cancer, and dementia. They lower cholesterol and triglycerides. And they are powerful anti-inflammatory compounds. But more important, they make your food tasty and satisfying.

In one dietary study in Spain, researchers split the study population into three groups. They were all told to eat a basic Mediterranean diet, but one group was given a liter of extra-virgin olive oil a week, another was given 30 grams (about an ounce) of nuts a day, and the

### Fighting Cholesterol

When Tracy Keibler started following The Daniel Plan, her cholesterol dropped. Her total cholesterol dropped from 260 to 207, with an LDL/HDL ratio of 1.6 and Total/HDL ratio of 2.5. Her triglycerides were 48. "All this happened without the use of a statin drug — or any drugs at all!" Tracy says. One of her doctors even told her she was a model patient. But that's not all.

"More significantly, my arsenal of medications is gone. I no longer require inhalers for asthma, my gastrointestinal issues are gone, and my eczema problems and sinus allergies are substantially better."

last group had only the diet. The groups who had the olive oil and nuts had over a 30 percent reduction in heart attacks and death.[2] This is a better result than statin drugs — without any of the side effects. More fat was better.

If you eat good quality fats with every meal, you will leave the table satisfied and without cravings. Your blood sugar will be balanced, and your brain will be happy. In fact, 60 percent of your brain is made from fat, specifically DHA. You can get DHA from fish and algae. Every one of your 10 trillion cells is wrapped in fatty membrane. The health of your cells determines your health, and the good fats make healthy cell membranes. (We discuss your brain health in chapter 6.)

We basically all need an oil change. Swap out the bad fats for the good and watch your health improve, your mood lift, your memory improve, and your skin, hair, and nails glow. So stock your pantry with a variety of healthy fats. Learn to use them. It can be as simple as grabbing a handful of nuts, opening a can of wild salmon, taking a spoonful of creamy coconut butter from the jar, or pouring extra-virgin olive oil (EVOO) over your veggies or salad.

Our favorite sources of good quality healing fats include foods we have already told you about. Fish and seafood are great sources of omega 3 fats (as well as protein and minerals). The best sources of omega 3 fats are sardines, herring, and wild salmon. Keep several cans in your pantry at all times. They are great on salad, or try them with a squirt of lemon and your favorite herb or spice. Nuts and nut butters (without added sugar, salt, or hydrogenated fats) provide monounsaturated fats. Make sure they are raw or lightly roasted. Grab a handful of nuts, or dip apple slices into a nut butter as a snack. Seeds are a fabulous food few people eat. They aren't just for birds.

Other healthy fats come from olives, avocados, and coconut. Olive oil and olives are rich in monounsaturated fats as well as antioxidant, anti-inflammatory polyphenol phytonutrients. Extra-virgin olive oil, cold-pressed, is the primary oil you should have on hand in your pantry. You can put it in salads or over vegetables, and cook with it on low to medium temperatures; at high temperatures it can oxidize and burn. For high-temperature cooking, use grape seed oil or coconut butter/oil. For flavor in cooking, such as in a stir fry, you can use unrefined sesame oil.

Avocados are a wonderful and unusual fruit that contain good monounsaturated fats and powerful anti-inflammatory compounds. Cut one in half and drizzle some balsamic vinegar on top. Put chopped avocados in salads, or mash them into guacamole with some lime juice, chopped tomatoes, diced onion, salt, and pepper. Avocados can make smoothies creamy and can even be used to make a healthy chocolate pudding. (Visit *danielplan.com* for the recipe "Amazing Avocado Gelato.")

Extra-virgin coconut butter or oil is an extraordinary super food that contains a special kind of anti-inflammatory saturated fat called lauric acid. It is the best source of the fuel your brain prefers, and it boosts your energy and brain power.

### Change Your Oil

Stock your pantry with the following unrefined oils that are good for your body and your brain:
- Extra-virgin olive oil (EVOO), cold-pressed: for dressings, marinades, and cooking over low to medium heat
- Extra-virgin coconut oil, cold-pressed or unrefined: for cooking even at medium high temperatures
- Grape seed oil: for cooking at higher temperatures
- 100% avocado oil: for cooking, less of this oil goes further than EVOO
- Sesame oil: for cooking when you want to add a bit of flavor

## WHAT ABOUT DRINKS?

We are going to have to tell you that your taste buds have been hijacked. Soda, sports drinks, flavored syrup-filled coffees, sweetened teas, juices, diet drinks, and energy drinks are super highways to obesity, cravings, and brain chemistry problems.

The single best and easiest thing you can do for your health is to recalibrate your taste buds and learn to enjoy pure clean water. You can add lemon or lime or herbs, have it sparkling or still, but you need about six to eight glasses of water a day.

Water should be your staple. The ideal water is filtered (to remove chlorine, pesticides, and other chemicals and bugs), comes from your tap, and is stored in a glass or stainless steel container.

Other drinks to enjoy if you want a little variety:

- *Herbal teas.* Simply put a few bags in a big glass jar, pour boiling water on top, let it steep, and then put in the fridge.

- *Green tea.* Plain iced green tea is a refreshing drink and packs a powerful healing punch.

- *Mint leaves, orange wedges, or cucumber slices.* Add them to your water for a little flavor.

- *Coffee.* A cup in the morning is an okay way to start the day, but too much coffee can raise your blood pressure and heart rate, increase anxiety, cause bone loss, and lead to even greater fatigue and insomnia. (See page 117 for more on coffee.)

## DON'T EVER BE IN
## A FOOD EMERGENCY AGAIN

We understand that busy lives make it challenging to find and eat good whole foods. We are on the go constantly. Every day, most Americans live in a constant state of busyness. They often skip breakfast or are at the mercy of the local coffee chain that offers high-sugar coffees and donuts or muffins or scones (which sound like a health food but are really giant sugar cookies in disguise). Then, at work there are bowls of candy and vending machines full of soda. On the way home, fast-food restaurants and convenience stores lure you in with a "quick fix" for your hunger. We live in a toxic nutritional wasteland, so the last place you want to find yourself is in a food emergency.

What is a food emergency? When your blood sugar starts to drop, you are hard-wired to eat anything (and everything) in sight. To think you can use willpower to control your hunger or cravings contradicts the science of how your brain controls your behavior. The more willpower you try to use, the more it backfires eventually. How often do you find yourself automatically overeating and bingeing, or just eating whatever happens to be in front of you?

But there is a solution — a simple, practical idea that most of us never think about: planning and bringing food with us. If you were a type 1 diabetic, you would not leave the house without your insulin syringe or a packet of sugar. If you did, your life would be at risk. If you had a severe peanut allergy, you wouldn't go anywhere without your Epi-pen. One sniff of peanut dust, and you could die without your protection.

While you may not die in an hour when you get hungry, you will get sick and fat and live a shorter, poorer life if you regularly find yourself in a food emergency. You will repeatedly choose poor quality, high sugar, refined foods and eat more than you need. A few things that will keep you from a food emergency include starting your day with a healthy balanced breakfast, eating every three to four hours, hydrating your body throughout the day, and stocking an emergency food kit.

We recommend that everyone create an emergency food pack; it will be your food safety net. Find your favorite things to include; the choices are plentiful. Stock these packs in your home, your travel bag or purse, your car, and your workplace with key rations for any food emergency. If you didn't have time to eat breakfast, what could you grab for the car? Or if you get busy at work, what can you find in your drawer to get you through the day, or what is at the ready in the late afternoon if you start to droop?

We recommend protein for many of the choices, because protein controls your appetite and balances your blood sugar over long periods

## Dr. Hyman's Go-To Travel Food Emergency Pack

When I am on the road, my health is in jeopardy every time I step out of my controlled environment. Airports, hotel mini-bars, and bad restaurants are often food deserts. So I bring food with me and make it a rule never to eat on planes or in airports (although increasingly you can find edible whole foods in airports; you just have to know how to hunt and gather!). I never leave home without these things, and I keep a good stock in my pantry, so I can just throw them in my bag. They take up little space and pack a powerful nutritional punch.

- Wild salmon jerky
- Grass-fed beef or turkey jerky
- Packets of coconut butter and macadamia nut butter
- Raw protein food bars
- Organic almonds
- Organic macadamia nuts
- Organic dates

of time. Protein snacks keep on giving, but without the quick rush and crash we get from most "snack foods" that leave us more hungry and tired. If you wait until you are hungry, you will make irrational decisions. So set yourself up to make better choices by having nutritious choices around you.

With a little bit of planning and shopping, we can stay healthy and out of food emergencies. Get a few glass containers with lids and sandwich baggies to put your snacks in. Buy an insulated lunch box or mini-cooler to put your food in. These are just ideas, and you can innovate, but make sure you include food with good quality protein, good fats, and low sugar content.

## Snack Items

Stock these items in your pantry; they keep forever:

- Canned wild salmon or sardines
- Flax or seed crackers
- Jerky (bison, grass-fed beef, or turkey)
- Salmon jerky
- Nuts and seeds
- Nut butter packets
- Coconut butter packets
- Whole food or raw food protein bars
- Artichoke hearts
- Roasted red peppers

Prepare a few easy, on-the-go snacks:

- Garbanzo beans with olive oil, lemon, garlic, and salt
- Hard-boiled eggs
- Hummus
- Cut-up carrots, cucumbers, peppers, and celery
- Apples or pears

It is also a good idea to stock a few treats:

- Dark chocolate (70%)
- Dried figs
- Dates

## WHAT ABOUT VITAMINS?

Overwhelming basic science and experimental data support the use of nutritional supplements for the prevention of disease and the support of optimal health. Vitamins don't work for everything, but they are critical for every chemical reaction and physiologic function of your body.

There are thousands of nutritional supplements on the market. Which ones should you take? Just trying to figure it out can be confusing, but it is actually quite simple. For most of us, a simple multivitamin and mineral, an omega 3 fat supplement, and vitamin D3 are all we need. There are other supplements that can benefit people as they age or for those with different conditions. You can read more about those online at *danielplan.com*.

## FOOD CRAVINGS AND ADDICTION

If I asked you to hold your breath underwater for fifteen minutes and promised to give you $1 million if you did it, could you do it? Of course not! We can't live without oxygen. Our brains are hardwired to crave it. Most of our brains also crave sugar. It is simply a survival mechanism. So if you believe willpower can rescue you from bad eating habits and cravings for junk food, sugar, or refined carbs, forget it. You might as well try to hold your breath for an hour.

It is a matter of hormones and brain chemistry. Fix those two things, and your cravings will go away in a couple of days (not for oxygen, though!). It is hard to imagine but true.

In the book *Salt Sugar Fat*, Michael Moss reveals that the food industry has intentionally and scientifically designed the hyper-processed, hyper-palatable, sugar-laden food to make us addicted — not metaphorically, but actually physically addicted. Think heroin lollipops or morphine muffins. The industry designed "craving experts" to find the "bliss point" of foods. Brain imaging studies confirm that these foods light up the parts of the brain that respond to opiates like heroin and stimulate hunger and cravings. In fact, sugar is more addictive than cocaine.[3] No wonder we have cravings!

## Tame the Four Hormones of the Apocalypse

It's easy to get your key hormones in balance. Here's how to cut the cravings:

- Cut out sugar and white flour. Go cold turkey.
- Cut out all artificial sweeteners.
- Increase fiber.
- Eat protein for breakfast.
- Eat a handful of nuts 15 minutes before a meal to cut your appetite.
- Stop night-time eating and bingeing.
- Focus on portion size. Learn appropriate portion sizes for lean proteins and whole grains.
- Wait 20 minutes before eating a second portion. It takes that long for food to hit the lower part of your small intestine and trigger PPY, the hormone that is a powerful brake on your appetite.
- Put your fork down between bites. It will slow you down, and by the time you get to seconds, you won't want any.
- Increase exercise, which you will read about in the next chapter.
- Sleep at least 7 to 8 hours a night. Those who lost even one or two hours of sleep a night craved more carbs and ended up eating more during the day.[4]
- Breathe. The simplest and fastest way to relax and reduce cortisol is to take five breaths. Count to five on the in breath, and count to five on the out breath. Do it five times.
- Play, which is a form of fitness, is something we do without thinking when we are young. It is a wonderful way to lower cortisol.
- Give and receive — one of the most powerful healing and restorative things in the world.

There are four key hormones that drive our brain chemistry and control our appetite and metabolism. We call these the "four hormones of the apocalypse." If you learn simple tricks to regain control of these hormones, your cravings will vanish quickly, usually in less than forty-eight hours. If you get these hormones under control, all the rest often resets automatically:

1. *Insulin* is produced in large quantities by the pancreas in response to sugar or starch that triggers fat storage in the belly and interferes with appetite control centers in the brain, making you hungry and craving more sugar and carbs.

2. *Ghrelin* is the hunger hormone produced in the stomach. Most of the ways we eat and live cause this hunger hormone to spike.

3. *PYY (peptide YY)* is produced in the intestine and puts the brakes on your appetite.

4. *Cortisol* is the stress hormone produced by the adrenal glands and during chronic stress causes hunger, storage of belly fat, and loss of muscle.

The beauty of adding food that heals, nourishes, and satisfies you deeply is that it will almost effortlessly shift your body and mind into a different state — a state where your cravings are gone, where your willpower is not needed because you naturally crave what makes you thrive and feel good. By adding simple habits — sleeping a bit more, moving your body, calming your mind, breathing, playing, serving — you will gradually, day by day, shift into a profound capacity for self-care and healing. Fulfillment, living with purpose, and well-being are the natural result.

Now that you have learned that food is medicine, that real food has the power to create a healthy life, and exactly what foods you can eat for the most powerful, life-giving energy, it is time to have a look at what we have been eating that we thought was food, but isn't, and how to avoid life-robbing, disease-promoting, obesity-inducing foods.

## The Cravings Stopped

Pastor Tom Crick had heard other people on The Daniel Plan say things like "You know, you will get over that after a little while. You'll stop craving sodas or sugar." *Yeah, right,* he thought.

As he focused on eating The Daniel Plan way, it started to change. "I found out that it's really true. I started to not crave those things anymore. I could taste the natural sugars in fruit and things like that.... Wow, a strawberry is really sweet! I never noticed before, because I was so used to artificial sugars."

# 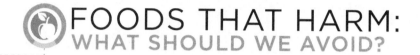 FOODS THAT HARM:
## WHAT SHOULD WE AVOID?

**JUST AS FOOD HAS THE POWER TO HEAL US,** it also has the power to harm us. The single biggest cause of our chronic disease epidemic, of a nation that is no longer thriving, is the poor quality of our food. It's hard to imagine that we feed ourselves and our children food that we wouldn't even feed our dog. Would you give your dog a cheeseburger, fries, and a soda? We hope not. Then why would you feed them to your kid? Why is there even such a thing as "kid's food" or a "kid's menu"? Guess what kids eat in Spain. Spanish food! What do kids eat in Indonesia? Indonesian food.

> "My house had only two things on the menu: take it, or leave it."
>
> — Dr. Hyman

We have been convinced that changing what we eat is hard. No wonder! In many communities in America there are ten times as many fast-food joints and convenience stores as supermarkets or produce markets. The average American consumes ten pounds of chemical additives a year. The more additives, typically the fewer the nutrients.

So we also want to educate you about the non-food or food-like substances that are hiding in the things we eat every day. Here's a simple way to know whether a food is non-food: If it takes longer to read and understand the label than to eat it, it's probably not food. If it has "ingredients" that your great-grandmother would not have used in cooking meals for her family, then likely it is not food.

Food contains calories, proteins, fats, carbohydrates, fiber, vitamins and minerals, phytonutrients, and plant genes where the sum of the whole food is far greater than any one ingredient. But over the last century, our food has been overthrown by anti-nutrients — food-like substances that often were never or have never been proven safe, such as chemically altered sugars; addictive, inflammatory super starches containing genetically transformed flour; processed fats, preserved with chemicals to make them last for years and colored with dyes to make them enticing. Factory foods are loaded with toxic fats, sugars, and salt.

These may seem convenient and inexpensive, but the real cost of eating these foods is depleting our health and human capital, not to mention what a chemically dependent agriculture system does to the environment. One pound of factory-farmed meat requires 2,000 gallons of water and produces 53 times as much greenhouse gases as a pound of vegetables.[5] (Both the Environment Working Group [*ewg. org*] and CleanFish [*cleanfish.com*] offer more information on how to reduce the environmental impact by intelligently choosing your food.) So what you eat is way more than just about your hungry stomach or your waistline. It affects everything!

## THE WHITE MENACES

One of the biggest threats to our health is the dramatic increase of sugar in all forms in our diet in the last hundred years. Hunter-gatherer populations consumed about 22 teaspoons of sugar a year; now the average American consumes 22 to 30 teaspoons of sugar every single day.[6] In 1800, the average person consumed 5 pounds per year;[7] now we average 152 pounds a year.[8] Our bodies are not designed to handle that amount of sugar. Paracelsus, the ancient Greek physician said, "The dose makes the poison." At the current dose, sugar is poison. The average 20-ounce soda has 15 teaspoons of sugar. Would you put that much in your cup of coffee or tea?

Sugar has many names: cane sugar, evaporated cane juice, brown sugar, dextrose, agave, maple syrup, honey, and of course, high fructose corn syrup (HFCS), which is now the single biggest source of calories in our diet. All of these are harmful when eaten in excess. Sugar-sweetened drinks like soda now make up 15 percent of the calories consumed by the average American. One can of soda a day increases a kid's risk of obesity by 60 percent and women's chance of getting diabetes by more than 80 percent.[9]

Other dangers are refined or processed white foods that spike blood sugar, but we don't think of them as sugar. They are white flour, white rice, and white pasta. These white foods act like sugar in the body. We should substitute with better options, such as bread made from whole kernel rye, or black or brown rice.

Since 1950, more than 600,000 packaged and processed foods have been introduced into the marketplace. Eighty percent of them are full of sugar, often tablespoons and tablespoons, hidden and disguised by all sorts of names.[10] It is in bread, ketchup, and salad dressings. In fact, the average serving of commercial spaghetti sauce has more sugar

## The Varieties of Sugar

### Familiar Sugars (not healthy, just real)

| | |
|---|---|
| Agave | Honey |
| Barley malt | Juice concentrate |
| Brown rice syrup | Maple syrup |
| Brown sugar | Molasses |
| Coconut sugar | Palm sugar |
| Evaporated or dehydrated cane juice | Sugar |

### Hidden Sugars or Toxic Sugars

| | |
|---|---|
| Dextrose | Glucose |
| Dextrin | Lactose |
| Disaccharides | Maltodextrin |
| Fructose | Maltose |
| High fructose corn syrup (or any corn sugar or syrup) | Monosaccharides |
| | Sorghum |
| Hydrogenated starch | Sucrose |
| | Xylose |

than a serving of chocolate sandwich cookies, which is why later in this chapter we will show you how to effectively read labels.

## WHY SUGAR IS THE MAIN CAUSE OF DISEASE

Since low-fat dietary recommendations in the early 1980s (which we all thought were good for us at the time), we have doubled our rates of obesity in adults and tripled it in kids, and the rate of type 2 diabetes around the world has increased sevenfold. In fact, today in America, one in two people have pre-diabetes or type 2 diabetes. We have seen the number of people with heart disease, type 2 diabetes, cancer, dementia, depression, and infertility skyrocket. (Actually, to diagnose cancer, doctors give patients radioactive sugar. The sugar then goes straight to the cancer, and it lights up on the PET scan.)

Sugar triggers a cascade of changes in your body that make you sick and fat. Here's what happens:

1. You eat quickly absorbed sugar or refined carbohydrates (like white flour).
2. Your blood sugar spikes.
3. Your insulin levels spike.
4. Insulin triggers the storage of belly fat and increases your appetite and sugar cravings.
5. The sugar (particularly the fructose in high fructose corn syrup) turns on a cholesterol factory in your liver (called lipogenesis), increasing LDL (bad cholesterol), lowering HDL (good cholesterol), and raising triglycerides.
6. This leads to a fatty liver (now affecting 60 to 90 million Americans).[11]

All of this increases something called *insulin resistance*, where your cells become numb to the effects of insulin, requiring more and more insulin to keep your blood sugar normal. This is the major cause of all age-related chronic disease (such as heart disease, high blood pressure, stroke, cancer, type 2 diabetes, and dementia.)

Your body makes more and more insulin, triggering more and more belly fat and inflammation. This inflammation is at the root of most chronic diseases. Whew! Even if someone doesn't yet have type 2 diabetes, insulin resistance is the major cause of heart attacks, strokes, many cancers, and even dementia (now called type 3 diabetes).

*Bottom line:* Sugar is an occasional treat. When you have sugar, stick with traditional, natural forms: raw sugar, raw honey, natural fruit sugars, pure maple syrup. Stay away from all the rest. Use it in things you make yourself, but sparingly, and use The Daniel Plan recipes on the website and in *The Daniel Plan Cookbook* as a guide to healthy desserts. Avoid all hidden and added sugars by carefully reading labels.

You can use whole fruit or fruit juices in small amounts as natural sweeteners in healthy desserts. As you start to eat real food, your cravings and addiction will be replaced by deep pleasure and satisfaction for naturally sweet things.

## Liquid Death: Don't Drink Your Calories

If there was one thing you could do to dramatically improve your health and lose weight, it would be this: Don't drink liquid sugar calories. This means soda, sports drinks, flavored coffees or teas, energy drinks, and juices (except fresh-made green vegetable juice).

Here's what liquid calories do:

- They get deposited and become that dreaded belly fat.
- They turn your liver into a fat factory triggering more insulin resistance and starting a vicious cycle.
- They mess with your head by increasing your appetite and keeping you from feeling full, so you eat more than you normally would in a day.

*Bottom line:* Stick to water or unsweetened, non-caffeinated teas.

## THE SPECIAL CASE OF FRUCTOSE

We can tolerate sugar in small amounts and as an occasional treat. One good source of sugar is real whole fruit (not juice or concentrate). The truth is, fructose that you get from eating fruit is fine because it is packaged in fiber and full of vitamins, minerals, and phytonutrients.

The problem is when the fructose is taken out of the fruit — which is how we get high fructose corn syrup (HFCS). Avoid HFCS at all costs. If you do nothing else to change your diet, make this one change and be relentless about it.

## ARTIFICIAL SWEETENERS

Since sugar causes so many health problems, why not switch to artificial sweeteners and diet foods made with these alternatives? If losing weight were all about the calories, then consuming diet drinks would seem like a good idea. A fourteen-year study of more than 65,000 women found that the opposite seems to be true. Diet drinks may be worse than sugar-sweetened drinks.[12]

There is no free ride. Diet drinks are not good substitutes for sugar-sweetened drinks. They also increase cravings, weight gain, and type 2 diabetes. And they are addictive. Watch for the hidden names of artificial or non-caloric or non-absorbed sweeteners such as aspartame, acesulfame, and sucralose; and sugar alcohols such as malitol and xylitol and anything else that ends in OL.

## WHAT ABOUT STEVIA?

Stevia seems like the perfect alternative to help avoid the dangers of artificial sweeteners such as aspartame. It comes from a plant. It's all natural. It has no calories. The Guarani Indians in Paraguay have used it since the sixteenth century. It sounds perfect. Until 1995 it was banned from the United States because of heavy lobbying by the makers of aspartame, an artificial sweetener. When the U.S. Food and Drug Administration (FDA) finally acted on it in 1995, it was approved as a dietary supplement sold in health food stores. This form of stevia is a good alternative.

However, read labels carefully, since some manufacturers have found a way to extract the bitter parts of the plant and keep just the sweet taste, turning what was potentially a better sweetener into a refined food substance. They isolated the sweet chemical called "rebauside A," or "reb A" for short.

Instead, go for the original whole plant extract, which you can find in health food stores or supermarkets. It comes in liquid or powder form. Keep in mind that sweets are treats, not staples.

As you follow The Daniel Plan, your taste buds will wake up to the wonderful taste of real food, you won't feel deprived, and your daily cravings will go away.

At this point you may be thinking you want to give up right now. *No sugar? Really?* The fact is, natural sugars found in fruit and some vegetables can taste incredibly sweet once you reclaim your taste buds. Life can still be very sweet without highly processed, refined sugars and artificial sweeteners. If you focus on real foods — foods that are naturally sweet such as fruit and even sweet vegetables — and learn to enjoy them, you won't miss the junk. And if you try junk again, it will taste extremely sweet. Try roasted vegetables or sweet potatoes. Even kids love them. Dark chocolate is also a wonderful treat in small amounts. There is always room for sweet treats in moderation.

## THE BAD FATS

The science of fat is so mixed up that it's no wonder everyone is confused. Thankfully, the new U.S. Dietary Guidelines are moving in the right direction, encouraging us to eat the right kinds of fats — which we already covered — and to avoid the bad ones.

There are two main classes of fats that are bad for us: trans fat, and processed and refined vegetable oils. Think of clear or yellow oils sold in big jugs used by most Americans and sold as vegetable, soybean, corn, or canola oil (previously called rapeseed and not a human food until recently). These are called omega 6 oils or polyunsaturated fats.

They are inflammatory. And by now, you know what inflammation leads to in your body!

Switch out these oils for ones that benefit your body and brain (see page 97). The exception is that you can use small amounts of unrefined oils — often called *cold-pressed* or *expeller-pressed* — such as from grape seeds, sesame seeds, or walnuts for cooking at home. And, of course, you can use extra-virgin olive oil and coconut oil.

Trans fats are poisons and, next to high fructose corn syrup, the most deadly ingredient in our food supply. There is no safe limit. There is no reason to ever eat them.

They are made in a factory where liquid vegetable oil (usually from soybeans) is chemically treated under high pressure to make it solid at room temperature. It improves shelf-life dramatically, which is why cookies can stay on the shelf for years and shortening is perfectly good to make piecrust from after thirty years in the cupboard. Yes, it improves shelf life. But do you know why they call it "shortening"? It shortens your life!

Trans fats increase your risk of the following health problems:

- Increased bad cholesterol and lower good cholesterol
- Risk of heart attack
- Obesity and type 2 diabetes
- Cancer
- Impaired brain functioning and dementia
- Increased inflammation

You will find trans fats in packaged baked goods, cookies, cakes, crackers, fried fast foods, chips, and popcorn. Walk down the aisle of any supermarket and try to find any food without "hydrogenated fat" on the nutrition label. Yes, trans fats are now labeled, but the food policy permits the label to say "zero trans fats" if the product has less than 2 grams per serving. Frozen whipped topping is made from water, hydrogenated fat, and high fructose corn syrup as the main ingredients, yet the label says "0 trans fats" because a serving has less than 0.5 grams. Call it legalized lying.

## How Does What We Eat Affect the Planet?

The things you put on your fork have the power to affect not only your health, but also agricultural practices, climate change, and even our economy. One church member told us about Nigerian farmers he met who were given seed by a large agricultural company at a cheaper price than their regular seed, but then the seeds from that crop couldn't be replanted. (They are designed that way.) The farmers then were forced to buy the seed from the same company at a higher price the next year and eventually couldn't afford to farm.

This pattern of industrial agricultural practices not only has impacted the quality of the food you eat, but also creates hunger in little children in Africa. When you stop buying industrial food, it has an enormous ripple effect. The power of your fork can change the world.

When it comes to our health and the health of the planet, we have a lot more to learn and study, but we don't need all the answers in order to take action. We can each make choices to buy more whole foods, sustainably raised animals, locally grown produce, and more. Just as we've learned that certain fats are good for us and others are destructive, we can learn what agricultural and food practices are best for us too.

## FACTORY-MADE SCIENCE PROJECTS

Other than getting rid of high fructose corn syrup and trans fat, the best thing you can do for your health is to avoid factory-made science projects with weird and strange molecules that haven't been made by God in nature.

Many common food additives cause everything from uncontrollable hunger and binge eating (blame MSG), to headaches, allergies, and damage to your gut. A few simple rules will protect you and your family from fake food substances.

**Eat under five.** Check a label for less than five ingredients that are all real foods such as tomatoes, water, and salt.

**Beware of MSG in all its hidden forms.** It not only causes headaches and brain fog, but is also used in animal experiments to induce overeating and bingeing in mice and rats to fatten them up to create an animal model to study obesity. MSG makes you hungry and binge, and it triples your insulin production, leading to storage of belly fat. Hidden names for MSG include...

- ☐ Any "flavors" or "flavoring"
- ☐ Anything containing "enzymes"
- ☐ Anything "enzyme modified"
- ☐ Anything "hydrolyzed"
- ☐ Anything with the word "glutamate" in it
- ☐ Autolyzed plant protein
- ☐ Autolyzed yeast
- ☐ Barley malt
- ☐ Bouillon and broth
- ☐ Carrageenan
- ☐ Gelatin
- ☐ Glutamate
- ☐ Glutamic acid sodium
- ☐ Hydrolyzed plant protein (HPP)
- ☐ Hydrolyzed vegetable protein (HVP)
- ☐ Malt extract
- ☐ Maltodextrin
- ☐ Monosodium glutamate
- ☐ Natural seasonings
- ☐ Protease
- ☐ Stock
- ☐ Textured protein
- ☐ Umami
- ☐ Vegetable protein extract
- ☐ Yeast extract
- ☐ Yeast food or nutrient

### What Am I Eating?

"I had to eat an MRE—meals ready to eat—while I was working after the earthquake in Haiti. When I read the label of the chicken and dumplings, there were more than 500 ingredients. I recognized almost none of them and couldn't pronounce most of them. In fact, I couldn't find chicken on the label—it was a 'chicken-like substance.'"

—Dr. Hyman

**Eat organic,** if you can afford it, to avoid pesticides, hormones, and antibiotics in food. If you are budget strapped, use the *Clean Fifteen* and *Dirty Dozen* list from the Environmental Working Group (*ewg. org*) to choose the least contaminated conventionally grown fruits and vegetables and avoid the most contaminated versions. Go to *ewg. org/agmag/2010/06/shoppers-guide-pesticides*. It is a bit more expensive, but being selective here can help the budget and your health. For dairy, we suggest buying organic and eating less. Organic foods have about 25 percent more nutrients than conventionally grown plant foods. Beef, poultry, and eggs are also items that are better for you if organic or sustainably raised. If more people used organics, the prices would come down.

**Eat sustainably.** Try to buy sustainably raised animals and animal products when you can. This will help you avoid pesticides, antibiotics, and hormones. Look for the terms *grass fed, pasture raised, free-range* or *organic,* or *made without hormones and antibiotics.* Ask your butcher where things come from and how they were raised.

## Avoid the Most Common Additives and Chemicals in Food

- ☐ MSG (monosodium glutamate)
- ☐ Artificial sweeteners
- ☐ Soy protein isolate (processed soy extract that causes cancer in animals)
- ☐ Sodium and calcium caseinate (toxic dairy extract)
- ☐ Phosphoric acid (dipotassium phosphate and tricalcium phosphate)
- ☐ Artificial flavors (often containing MSG)
- ☐ Carrageenan (can cause leaky gut and inflammation)
- ☐ Colors and dyes (yellow dye #5 or tartrazine and others)
- ☐ Sulfites (cause allergies and inflammation)
- ☐ Nitrites and nitrates (in processed and deli meats and causes cancer)

## WHAT ABOUT CAFFEINE?

Most Americans, along with millions of people around the world, love coffee. It is made from coffee beans, a plant food. There are pros and cons of coffee.

**The Cons:**

- Increases stress hormones, anxiety, and irritability
- Increases blood pressure and heart rate
- Increases insulin
- Being addictive, can cause headaches in withdrawal
- Interferes with sleep and causes insomnia
- Can cause acid reflux and heartburn
- Can cause palpitations
- Can cause loss of minerals, such as magnesium and calcium, in the urine
- Being a diuretic, can cause dehydration
- Causes short-term energy but increases fatigue later

**The Pros:**

- Increases focus and concentration
- Enhances sports performance
- Can help constipation
- May be linked to lower risk of prostate cancer, dementia, stroke, and heart failure
- May lower risk of diabetes
- Smells good and tastes great

*Bottom line:* If you enjoy a cup of coffee in the morning, enjoy it. But we are talking real, fresh coffee — not the sugar and dairy-laden large mocha latte. Be mindful of what you put in it, and we recommend no more than one to two cups a day. Everyone has a different tolerance and response to coffee. Notice yours. The only exception is that we encourage you to try The Daniel Plan Detox recalibration.

That's when we suggest you avoid stimulants and sedatives to see how you really feel. (See page 294 for information on the detox plan.)

## What about Alcohol?

Wine, beer, and spirits have been around almost as long as the human race. But it is controversial for moral, personal, and medical reasons.

Be aware that in doses of more than one or two glasses, alcohol becomes a poison, and it is a source of high calories and sugar that can significantly contribute to weight gain. Too much alcohol causes damage to your gut lining, damages your liver, and increases blood sugar and insulin. It can also cause inflammation, disrupt hormones, cause brain atrophy, and deplete your vitamin levels. One glass may bring health benefits, but more than two can bring harm.

Unfortunately, alcohol addiction is common and robs people and their families of their lives. For those with addiction or prone to addiction, abstinence is the best medicine. (If someone you love is struggling with an alcohol addiction, you can find out how to help them at *celebraterecovery.com*.) Also, if you have a high risk of breast cancer, are prone to mental illness, have liver or digestive problems, have a personal or family history of alcoholism, or are allergic to sulfites in wine, then you shouldn't consume any alcohol.

## FOOD SENSITIVITIES AND ALLERGIES

The old saying goes that what is one man's medicine is another man's poison. Nowhere is this truer than when it comes to our different responses to food. And nowhere in medicine is there more controversy, superstition, and confusion than there is surrounding the subject of food allergies, sensitivities, and illness.

As a doctor in active medical practice, Dr. Hyman has had at his disposal two powerful medicines for treating, reversing, and even curing hundreds of diseases. These medicines are (1) addressing hidden food sensitivities and food allergies, and (2) getting people to eat real foods. The science of functional medicine (his specialty) is about connecting the dots and treating your body as a holistic system, not just focusing on symptoms.

The two most common foods that trigger reactions are gluten (found in wheat, barley, rye, spelt, and oats) and dairy. These foods trigger inflammation, which is the root of autoimmune diseases (suffered by 24 to 50 million Americans);[13] arthritic, allergic, and asthmatic diseases, which are all on a steep rise; diabetes; dementia; obesity; depression; heart disease; and autism.

So why are we seeing an epidemic of inflammatory disease in this country? Is it a sudden genetic mutation that has millions of us overreacting to foods we have apparently eaten for thousands of years?

The answer is no.

We have to start looking for delayed or hidden food reactions that cause inflammation. These reactions might be hard to detect. If you eat bread on Monday, you might get a migraine on Wednesday, or just generally feel bloated, or have brain fog, or gain weight and become pre-diabetic. The symptoms can be vague: fatigue, bloating, brain fog, food cravings, sinus congestion or post nasal drip, acne, eczema, psoriasis, irritable bowels, acid reflux, headaches, joint pains, trouble sleeping, asthma, and more.

The food allergies we are referring to are different. They are low-grade reactions that cause problems over a long period of time and lead to chronic rather than acute illnesses. These may affect up to 50 percent of the population.

There are blood tests for these reactions, and if you are concerned that you have a serious gluten sensitivity or celiac disease, you should get the proper blood tests. However, for most of us a two-to-six-week trial of eliminating these foods will tell you more than any tests. Your body has infinite wisdom. Listen to it. What symptoms get better? How do you feel? Do you lose weight?

The rise of these food sensitivities now is directly related to what we've been eating. Our processed, low-fiber, high-sugar diet alters the bacteria that live in our digestive system. You have 500 species of bugs in there. The bacteria outnumber your cells 10 to 1, and you have 100 times more bacterial DNA in you than your own DNA. What research shows is the existence of "leaky gut," where food proteins leak across a damaged intestinal lining and activate your immune system. When you eat processed food, you change your gut flora and foster the

## What about Dairy?

Americans have been taught that we need milk, that without it kids will not grow up to be big and strong and old ladies' bones will dissolve in a heap from osteoporosis. We have been taught that milk is nature's perfect food. It is. For a calf! Humans are the only species that drinks milk after weaning. More than 75 percent of the world's population is lactose intolerant (having the inability to digest the sugar in milk), and dairy causes bloating, gas, and diarrhea. Beyond lactose intolerance, the adverse immune responses to the proteins in dairy abound, including congestion, asthma, sinus problems, kids' ear infections, rashes and eczema, autoimmune diseases, and type 1 diabetes. We encourage everyone to take a dairy holiday and eliminate dairy for at least ten days but up to forty days to see how you feel. Along with gluten (see p. 122), dairy is one of the most inflammatory foods in our diet.

Some people may tolerate dairy in small amounts. If you want to include dairy and find that you tolerate it, here is how to minimize your risk:

- Try sheep or goat milk or cheese.
- Choose dairy products that are organic and from pasture-raised animals.
- Stick with hard cheeses rather than processed cheeses.
- Use more easily digested forms of dairy such as kefir or plain yogurt, which contain beneficial bacteria.

growth of bad bugs that promote inflammation. Add to that the gut-busting drugs we use — antibiotics, anti-inflammatories, acid blockers, and steroids — combined with our stressful lives, and we have the perfect environment for a leaky gut.

Then you get a stomach flu or traveler's diarrhea or take one more course of antibiotics, and — wham! — suddenly you get a leaky gut. Your immune system (60 percent of which lies right under your intestinal lining) gets exposed to food and bacterial particles. Your normal balance is disrupted. You can't digest food properly or determine friend from foe, and your immune system creates an abnormal reaction to something pretty normal — the food you eat.

## WHAT YOU CAN DO TO HEAL

We can do many things to deal with delayed food allergies or sensitivities, rebalance our systems, and get rid of our chronic symptoms.

Here are a few things you can do to heal your leaky gut:

1. For ten to forty days, stop eating gluten and dairy 100 percent. Even 99 percent won't do the trick. Your immune system responds to microscopic things. We designed The Daniel Plan Detox to give you a meal plan that cuts out dairy and gluten (see page 294).

2. After you have been off those foods for ten to forty days, add one back in every three days and monitor your symptoms in *The Daniel Plan Journal* to track what causes symptoms that can be delayed by two-to-forty-eight hours after eating the food.

3. Take a probiotic (healthy beneficial bacteria) to help regulate your immune system. Look for brands in the health food store or online from reputable sources that contain a mixture of beneficial bacteria, including Lactobacillus rhamnosus and Bifidobacterium, with at least 30 to 50 billion organisms per dose. Foods that contain probiotics include sauerkraut, kimchi, miso or tempeh, and kombucha. Unsweetened yogurt and kefir are fine if you are not sensitive to dairy.

4. Add more fiber to your diet (see page 81).

5. Digestive enzymes help break down food and make it less likely to cause an allergic reaction. Look for broad-spectrum enzymes that contain proteases, amylases, and lipases. They can be either plant or animal derived. There are natural enzymes in your digestive tract, which is how you break down food, but when you have a leaky gut, they may not work as well.

6. Take a good multivitamin and fish oil (1 to 2 grams a day, certified free of metals and other toxins), which contains nutrients that help the digestive system heal.

7. Other nutrients can be helpful to heal a leaky gut, including zinc, vitamin A, evening primrose oil, and glutamine.

If problems persist, consider testing for IgG allergens with a blood test and working with a doctor trained in dealing with food allergies. (See *functionalmedicine.org* to find a doctor trained in Functional Medicine.)

## IS WHEAT DANGEROUS? THE PROBLEM WITH GLUTEN

The heirloom biblical wheat of our ancestors is something modern humans never eat. Instead, we eat dwarf wheat, the product of genetic manipulation and hybridization, that created short, stubby, hardy, high-yielding wheat plants with much higher amounts of starch and gluten. The man who engineered this modern wheat won the Nobel Prize because it promised to feed millions of starving people around the world. Well, it has. But it brought some issues with it.

> The average American eats 146 pounds of flour a year.[14]

This type of wheat also contains special forms of a protein called *gluten*, the glue-like protein that makes dough sticky. Gluten is found in wheat barley, rye, spelt, oats, and kamut and holds bread together and makes it rise. The dwarf wheat grown in the United States has changed the quality and type of gluten proteins in wheat, creating much higher gluten content, and creating a super-gluten that causes celiac disease and autoimmune antibodies.

Combine this with the damage our guts have suffered from our diet, environment, lifestyle, and medications, and now you know why gluten intolerance is on the rise. This super gluten crosses our leaky guts and gets exposed to our immune system. Our immune system reacts as if gluten is something foreign, and it sets off the fires of inflammation in an attempt to eliminate it. However, this inflammation is not selective, so it begins to attack our cells.

Low-level inflammation from gluten that is not celiac disease has been shown to increase heart attacks by more than 35 percent and cancer by more than 70 percent.[15] That is why elimination of gluten and food allergens or sensitivities can be a powerful way to prevent and reverse obesity, diabetes, and so many other chronic diseases.

### Gluten-Free Worked for Me

On a visit to Saddleback Church, Dr. Hyman talked about how you could be following the principles of The Daniel Plan and still feel unwell. So if that was the case, you should try going off gluten. When Cindy Sproul heard him say that, she perked up. "A little bell went off in my head. *That's why I'm still not feeling well*, I thought. I had been having migraine headaches probably weekly for three or four years. That day, I went off gluten and within three days, I didn't have a headache left.

"I was thinking clearer. I didn't have stiffness and swelling in my hands and joints. I had more energy and felt reignited."

*Bottom line:* If you have any chronic illness, are overweight, or just want to see how good you can feel, try a gluten-free diet for ten to forty days. It is a powerful way to identify the cause of chronic health problems. Combined with dairy elimination, it can cure many diseases, accelerate weight loss, and renew your body and mind.

## THE DANIEL PLAN DETOX

We recommend that everyone start with a ten-day (which you can extend to forty days) Daniel Plan Detox to jump-start the healing process, reboot your system, and discover the power of reclaiming your body and mind by letting go of the things that can harm you and adding in the things that can heal you. Using the power of healing foods, your body and mind will quickly transform, and you will realize just how well you can feel and how quickly it can happen.

### Why Should I Do The Daniel Plan Detox?

Many of us usually feel less than fully healthy. We either have nagging complaints such as fatigue and brain fog or more serious illnesses. By giving your body a chance to reset for a short period of time, you will learn firsthand the power of food to heal and the abundance, energy, and vibrancy that can come from a healing way of eating.

Here are the benefits you can experience in just a few weeks:

- Weight loss of 5 – 10 pounds or more
- Better digestion and elimination
- Fewer symptoms of chronic illness
- Improved concentration, mental focus, and clarity
- Improved mood and increased sense of internal balance
- Increased energy and sense of well-being
- Less congestion and fewer allergic symptoms
- Less fluid retention
- Less joint pain
- Increased sense of peace and relaxation
- Enhanced sleep
- Improved skin

It is as simple as taking out the bad stuff and putting in the good stuff. Dr. Hyman and Dr. Amen have seen patients recover from a long list of chronic diet-related symptoms and diseases quickly, problems they had never before connected to what they were eating. If you have any of these symptoms or diseases, consider doing The Daniel Plan Detox for ten days or extending it to forty days.

- ☐ Arthritis
- ☐ Autoimmune diseases
- ☐ Bad breath
- ☐ Bloating, gas, constipation, or diarrhea
- ☐ Canker sores
- ☐ Chronic fatigue syndrome
- ☐ Diabetes or pre-diabetes
- ☐ Difficulty concentrating
- ☐ Excess weight or difficulty losing weight
- ☐ Fatigue
- ☐ Fibromyalgia
- ☐ Fluid retention
- ☐ Food allergies
- ☐ Food cravings
- ☐ Headaches and migraines
- ☐ Heartburn
- ☐ Heart disease
- ☐ Inflammatory bowel disease (Crohn's or ulcerative colitis)
- ☐ Irritable Bowel Syndrome
- ☐ Joint pain
- ☐ Menopausal symptoms (mood changes, sleep problems, hot flashes)
- ☐ Menstrual problems (premenstrual syndrome, heavy bleeding, cramps)
- ☐ Migraines
- ☐ Muscle aches
- ☐ Puffy eyes and dark circles under the eyes
- ☐ Sinus congestion
- ☐ Postnasal drip
- ☐ Skin rashes (eczema, acne, psoriasis)
- ☐ Sleep problems

The Daniel Plan Detox includes the fundamentals laid out in the entire Daniel Plan: faith, food, fitness, focus, and friends. The only difference is that for a short time you stop anything that could potentially trigger health issues. Even if you think you don't have a problem, you might see a big difference. If a horse has been standing on your foot your whole life, then you may not know how bad it feels until he gets off your foot. Most of Dr. Hyman's patients say, "Dr. Hyman, I didn't know I was feeling so bad until I started feeling so good!" That is our prayer for all of you.

### Eating Away the Pain

"The Daniel Plan was really pretty simple, but at first not easy," Latrice Sarver recalls. "I had developed so many bad food habits and had yo-yo dieted for my entire life, there was a lot that I needed to change.

"I never dreamt that my pain would be affected in any way. When we did the detox at the very beginning, I soon discovered that I had decreased pain when I avoided animal protein and that my pain increased significantly when I added it back into my diet. By focusing primarily on fruits, vegetables, seeds, nuts, and whole grains, I had so much less pain, improved energy, improved blood sugars, and gradual weight loss."

We hope you will give yourself the gift of this powerful healing kick-start to The Daniel Plan. Real food, infused with spices and cooked or prepared, simply tastes far better than any processed food. It may take a week or two to reclaim your taste buds, but they will come back! And you will start to crave real, fresh food. Yes, really!

# 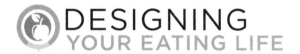DESIGNING
## YOUR EATING LIFE

**NOW THAT YOU HAVE LEARNED** what to eat and what to avoid, how can you make the shift? The sad reality is that it's easy to eat poorly. Health is not something that happens automatically. We are very good at planning for some areas of our life: vacation, parties, and maybe our financial future. But most of us rarely plan for our health.

Eating for health takes some work at first, but once you know the basics, you can be mindful and intentional pretty easily. Start by setting up your environment so that healthy choices are not just easy, but automatic. The Daniel Plan sets you up for success so that after forty days, you won't even have to think twice about it being your ongoing lifestyle. The key is to design your life to succeed. You will be ready for all that God has planned for you.

Imagine if at any time you were hungry, the food that nourishes and heals and satisfies you was right there at hand. Imagine if you knew exactly how to manage eating when on the road or when eating out or just surviving the average day at work.

With food, we will show you how to design your eating life for success, how never to be in a food emergency, how to shop and read labels, how to eat well for less, how to remake your pantry, kitchen, and freezer, a few simple cooking ideas, and even ideas for growing some of your own food. You will learn how to make your home, work, social life, and even the neighborhood safe food environments.

> The idea of designing your life applies to all the Essentials. Living life The Daniel Plan way takes you on a journey to restore not only your physical health, but your spiritual, mental, and relational health as well.

Before you change anything, it is a brilliant idea to start using *The Daniel Plan Journal*. Write down everything you eat: portion size, type of food, time, how you feel when eating it (stressed, hungry, bored, fatigued). Writing down what you eat does two things: It makes you conscious of what you really are eating, and it helps you shift and change your habits. Share your journal with your friends, buddy, or small group. You will learn a lot about yourself, and as you do, you will be able to easily make changes that bring healing to your body and mind. If you would rather use a virtual journal, download The Daniel Plan App.

> People who keep food journals lose twice as much weight as those who don't.[16]

## DESIGN YOUR KITCHEN

Health starts in the home — in fact, in the kitchen. You have to do a makeover of your kitchen. You may need to learn a few cooking skills. Most Americans spend more time watching cooking on television than actually cooking. We think that it is difficult and time consuming. Soon you will see that that is just a myth.

So it is time to have an honest look into the cupboards, keep all the good stuff, and dump the bad. Get out your magnifying glass.

### KITCHEN MAKEOVER: THINGS TO REMOVE

Start with things you should throw in the garbage because they should never be eaten by any human or any other living thing. There is a reason that flies won't land on a tub of margarine. If a fly wouldn't even eat it, should you? Look in your fridge, freezer, and pantry to identify processed foods, containing any of these three ingredients: high

### Pantry Makeover

Watch Dr. Amen and his wife, Tana, make over someone's pantry. Go to *danielplan.com* to watch the video "What Is in Your Pantry?"

fructose corn syrup, trans fat, and monosodium glutamate (MSG) — which you've already learned about in this chapter.

Also take an inventory of the packaged foods you have. There are colors, dyes, additives, nitrates, and other chemicals in most packaged foods. There are alternatives to your favorite foods in the average grocery store. It will take a little detective work, but learning to be a smart label reader is one of the most important things you can do for your health and the health of your family.

### KITCHEN MAKEOVER: THINGS TO ADD

Start a shopping list of pantry staples that you should always have on hand. Pick and choose items based on your taste preferences, but don't be afraid to try new foods.

#### CANS OR JARS

- ☐ Artichoke hearts
- ☐ Beans (black, garbanzo, cannellini, lentils, etc.)
- ☐ Coconut milk
- ☐ Curry paste
- ☐ Herring or mackerel
- ☐ Roasted red peppers
- ☐ Sardines
- ☐ Salsas
- ☐ Tomatoes, tomato sauce and paste
- ☐ Wild salmon

#### BAGS

- ☐ Bags of different nuts (pecans, walnuts, almonds, cashews, pine nuts, hazelnuts, Brazil nuts)
- ☐ Bags of jerky (organic, grass-fed beef, turkey, or bison with no nitrates or MSG)
- ☐ Bags of seeds (pumpkin, sesame, sunflower, flax, chia, hemp)

#### BOTTLES

- ☐ Balsamic vinegar
- ☐ Chicken or vegetable broth (low sodium)
- ☐ Healthy oils (extra-virgin olive, coconut, grape seed, avocado, and/or sesame)
- ☐ Sesame oil for flavoring (dark or light)
- ☐ Wheat-free tamari (soy sauce)

## BULK ITEMS

☐ Beans (lentils, garbanzo, black, cannellini, white beans, adzuki beans)

☐ Whole grains (brown, black, and red rice; quinoa; buckwheat)

## SPICES

☐ Bay leaves

☐ Black pepper (whole peppercorns and a grinder)

☐ Cinnamon

☐ Chili peppers

☐ Chili powder

☐ Coriander

☐ Cumin

☐ Oregano

☐ Red chili flakes

☐ Rosemary

☐ Turmeric

☐ Sea salt

## NUT BUTTERS (without added sugars or fat)

☐ Almond butter

☐ Coconut butter

☐ Macadamia nut butter

## SWEETENERS

☐ Raw honey, pure maple syrup, raw sugar

☐ Whole plant extract stevia

## CONDIMENTS AND SAUCES

☐ Fruit spreads (only 100% fruit, no sugar)

☐ Hot sauce (choose different varieties)

☐ Kimchi (spicy fermented cabbage)

☐ Mustard (coarse or Dijon)

☐ Miso paste

☐ Natural ketchup (no high fructose corn syrup)

☐ Sauerkraut

☐ Tahini (sesame paste)

☐ Tomato sauce

## EVERYDAY INGREDIENTS

Having the right things on hand equips you to succeed and is essential to your culinary success. Of course, the foundation of your basic pantry is complemented by an abundance of fresh, real, whole foods, but there are some *everyday ingredients* that will save you in a pinch and ensure that you are prepared to put together a quick, healthy meal in a matter of minutes.

> Stock your kitchen with everyday foods — namely, an abundance of fresh, non-starchy vegetables, lean protein, beans and legumes, whole grains, and seasonal fresh fruit.

### CHOPPED VEGETABLES

Choose your chopping time and be ready for healthful snacking anytime. Fresh, raw veggies pair deliciously with hummus, guacamole, and salsa and amplify your dose of nourishing food. Cut up the classics such as carrots and celery, but give some others a try, such as red peppers, cucumbers, cauliflower, and snap peas. If you are feeling adventurous, try jicama, a Mexican standard that is a good source of fiber.

### FRESH GREENS

Because they are a must for every vibrant kitchen, explore the wide array of greens at your local market, from the classic, well-loved baby spinach to lacinto kale and collards. Fresh greens provide your body with an abundance of nutrients that boost your energy and literally take your eating lifestyle up to a whole new level. Grab a handful to complement your morning smoothie, make your own custom mix of greens for salads, or sauté them with a little extra-virgin olive oil and fresh garlic. Your taste buds will explode! *Bottom line:* You can never have too many greens.

### BERRIES

Make berries the star of your smoothie and invite them into your morning oatmeal and as an embellishment to salads. An economical way to go organic is to buy frozen organic berries. Blueberries are one of Dr. Amen's top fifty brain foods and contain vital antioxidants.

Strawberries are packed with vitamins, fiber, and high levels of antioxidants.

## AVOCADO

Keep your kitchen stocked with delicious and nutritious avocados on a daily basis.

## ALTERNATIVE MILKS

Many people have discovered they are sensitive to dairy, and if you are one of them, say hello to your new best friend — almond milk. This wonderful, nourishing liquid is a blessing in your kitchen and can be used wherever you would have previously used dairy milk. Use it as the base for your morning smoothie. If you are a coffee drinker, try an almond milk latte. Another milk alternative is hemp or coconut milk; be sure to buy the unsweetened kind.

### Homemade Hummus

Start buying garbanzo beans and tahini. This dynamic duo sets you up for success. Having them on hand equips you to make your own hummus in a snap. In a blender or food processor, mix the following:

2 cans of garbanzo beans (buy organic if you can)

2 tablespoons tahini

6 tablespoons of extra-virgin olive oil

2 teaspoons ground cumin

Juice from one lemon

1 teaspoon salt

Dash or two of ground pepper

Get the texture you like by adding in a little warm water to blend. Have fun experimenting by adding in fresh minced garlic or your favorite herbs. This will become a mainstay in your kitchen portfolio.

## DESIGN YOUR WORKSPACE

Most of us live our lives in a fairly small circumference: home, work, church, friends, neighborhood. It's where we spend most of our time. That is why it's important to design your life for success. If you had a GPS tracker on you and could watch where you spend 90 percent of your time, you would be surprised. That is why setting up your work environment for success is key.

Whether you work at home, work in an office, or travel around in your car, designing your work life to include real, fresh, whole food — knowing what to bring, where to shop, or where to eat in your immediate area — is essential for success. There is free or cheap processed food everywhere at work: donuts, bagels, candy jars, sodas. And most likely, fast-food restaurants surround you.

The solution is easy. Get your emergency food pack (see page 98) together and have a version for home, for work, for your car, for your travel bag. If you start to get hungry, have something. If you wait until you are starving, you will overeat. Grab a handful of nuts, a piece of jerky, a packet of nut butter. You will feel better and do better! If you do crave something sweet, have a piece of fruit or a piece of dark chocolate.

Some other simple ideas can make being at work healthier:

*Have a lunch club.* Find a group of five to ten co-workers and agree to have one person bring in lunch for everyone once a week or every two weeks. You get real fresh food and only have to make something once every month or two.

*Create a salad club.* Get a group from work to sign up to bring salad ingredients to work once a week. Keep them in the fridge, and share. Post a checklist of salad ingredients such as greens (no iceberg lettuce), crunchy option (carrots, cucumbers), protein (nuts, hard-boiled eggs, or canned salmon), and items for homemade dressing such as balsamic vinegar, extra-virgin olive oil, Dijon mustard, and ground pepper; or extra-virgin olive oil, lime juice, cumin, and cayenne.

*Find a Daniel Plan buddy.* If you are doing The Daniel Plan through your church or on your own, it is still essential to try to find a buddy at work or in your neighborhood who can do it with you. (We will cover this more in chapter 7.) Getting healthy is a team sport, and being accountable to someone else and helping motivate and being motivated by a partner can double your success and make the changes stick.

## DESIGN YOUR SOCIAL LIFE

Part of life is going out and being with friends, going to events, eating at restaurants, and traveling. The good news is, you can eat almost anything occasionally and be fine — as long as it's real food, such as real pizza or French fries (not fast-food fries that have about thirty ingredients) or a piece of cake or cookies, and as long as you or someone you know made them from real ingredients.

So if 90 percent of the time you eat well, you can have treats and party food 10 percent of the time. To stay focused on eating well and still enjoying a vibrant social life, here are some basic strategies:

*Never go to a party hungry.* If you have a snack before, you won't be tempted to eat every greasy, fried, or sugary food.

*Eat before you travel.* Never go to an airport, a ball game, or a public event hungry.

*Bring your food.* If you are going to a picnic, bring healthy choices to eat if there is nothing else worth eating.

*Start a trend with your friends.* See who can find the best real food in your town. You can read menus online and make sure there are healthy choices.

*Stock up on the road.* If you are traveling, stock up on healthy snacks or restock your emergency food pack.

*Start a supper club with your friends or church group.* Rotate hosting the meal once a month between friends. Do a potluck or cook recipes from The Daniel Plan, which are available online (in The Daniel Plan App) and in *The Daniel Plan Cookbook*.

*Say no to food pushers.* These are people who say, "Come on, just have one bite" or "One can of soda can't hurt you." They might feel bad about themselves and want you to join. But have more respect for yourself and just say, "No thanks!"

## ENJOYING RESTAURANTS

Eating out is one of life's great pleasures. A server treats you like a king or queen. No fuss. No washing dishes. Our overall suggestion is to eat out less often and choose higher quality food when you do go out. When you go out, enjoy great food and feel great too. Here's how to eat well, feel well, and have fun eating out while still following The Daniel Plan.

*Look online before you get in line.* Check out menus online and look for healthy choices, good quality protein, simple dishes, sides of vegetables, clues such as *local, seasonal, organic, grass fed* on the menu, as well as gluten- or dairy-free options, which are becoming more common. Try apps like Google Plus or Yelp to see how restaurants are rated and what they serve; type in the words *organic, natural foods, vegetarian, slow food,* or *whole foods.*

*Try ethnic restaurants* such as Thai, Japanese, and Indian that use fresh ingredients. Sometimes they add a lot of sugar, fat, and salt, or even MSG, so you have to be discerning with their menus.

*Be annoying.* You can ask for substitutions or changes.

*Skip the bread.* Don't let them put bread and butter on the table.

*Avoid drinking alcohol __before__ you eat.* Alcohol makes you hungrier and less inhibited.

*Drink water,* at least a glass or two, before you eat. You will likely eat less.

*Skip the white sides,* and ask for extra vegetables.

*Order two or three sides of veggies.* Go crazy!

*Dress yourself.* Ask for extra-virgin olive oil, vinegar, and fresh pepper for your salad instead of dressings.

*Think about the perfect plate.* How can you order to have a smaller protein and starch portion and more veggies? Have salads and sides of veggies, share an entrée. Skip the white flour, white rice, and white potatoes.

*Avoid foods associated with certain words,* such as *glazed, fried, crispy, breaded,* and *creamy.*

*Choose foods associated with good words,* such as *roasted, broiled, baked, grilled, seared, steamed,* and *sautéed.*

*If eating breakfast out,* order the omelets or two poached eggs over steamed spinach and skip the white toast. You can ask for a bowl of berries.

*Share one dessert with the table* or order one that contains real fruit, is 70 percent cacao, and is free of refined sugars.

*Skip the appetizer.*

*Follow the "hari hachi bu" rule.* The Okinawans from Japan live well over 100 years old and eat until they are 80 percent full.

*Eat on time.* Don't go into a restaurant really hungry. You will order and eat more. Have a handful of almonds before you go. Eat three meals a day at regular intervals to balance your blood sugar and hormones.

*Bring leftovers home.* If the restaurant has large portions, ask for half the meal to be packed up before you even start eating. You will have lunch for tomorrow.

*Share entrées with a friend or companion.* Often portions are double what a normal person should eat.

*Be mindful.* Slow, conscious eating will allow you to really taste your food and your body to register that it is actually full — which takes twenty minutes from your first bite.

## DESIGN YOUR MIND

There are two reasons to be mindful when you eat. First, you will eat less and enjoy your food more. Second, you will metabolize and burn food better rather than store it in your belly. Study after study shows that when we eat unconsciously, we eat more.[17] In one study, participants were given snack food bags that automatically refilled from a secret compartment under the table. They were compared to folks who just had a single bag full. The group that had the auto-refillable bags just kept eating.[18] If you have a bigger plate, you will put more on it and eat more than if you had a smaller plate. If you savor every bite, you will eat less because you will enjoy your food more. Have you ever mindlessly finished a giant bag of buttered popcorn at the movies and then felt sick afterward? We have!

Studies also show that when you eat in a stressed state, you store fat in your belly and don't metabolize your food well. Same food, but more weight gain and inflammation.[19]

Eating is a sacred, wonderful experience that can connect you to your senses, your body, and the extraordinary flavors in real food. One of Dr. Hyman's patients said he wanted to lose weight but couldn't change his lunchtime habit of two big cheeseburgers that he ate in the car before he got out of the parking lot. Rather than telling him to stop eating the burgers, Dr. Hyman suggested that he simply go inside the restaurant, sit down, breathe deeply, close his eyes, and savor every single bite. At his next appointment he told Dr. Hyman that he never would eat a fast-food burger again, because when he really tasted it, he realized he actually didn't like it.

Are you starting to see how your mind can make such a big difference in your eating habits? That is why focus, the topic of chapter 6, is so important. There are a few simple things you can do to eat more mindfully, get more pleasure from food, and design your habits, your environment, and your mind to work on autopilot so that after a while you don't have to think about what you are doing. You will naturally just do the right thing.

*Say a blessing of thanks before each meal.* Gratitude and prayer honor God and help focus the mind and bring you to the present moment.

*Always sit down and sit still.* While eating, eat! Skip watching TV, talking on the phone, driving, standing, or walking down the street with food in your mouth. In Europe you can't actually get a to-go coffee; coffee is served only in ceramic cups at tables or the espresso bar.

*Eat from smaller plates.* Eating out of a package, bag, or container is a sure way to overeat and eat unconsciously. Use a 10-inch plate or bowl whenever you can.

*Stop and breathe before eating.* Take five deep breaths in and out through your nose before every meal.

*Create a peaceful environment.* Soft light, candles, quiet music, flowers. Any of these encourage attention, slow eating, and pleasure, all of which will lead you to eat less — as much as 18 percent less![20]

*Start with healthy foods first.* Starting with a salad or grilled veggies will lead you to eat less.

*Chew each bite multiple times.* You will improve digestion of your food and your enjoyment of it.

*Serve food before you put the plate on the table.* Leave the serving dish on the counter rather than in the center of the dining table.

*Don't reward exercise* by thinking, *I just walked 3 miles, so I can have a [fill in the blank].* Exercise is its own reward. Plus, if you have one 20-ounce soda, you have to walk 4.5 miles to burn it off. If you eat one super-sized meal, you have to run 4 miles a day for one week to burn off that one meal. You can't exercise your way out of a bad diet.

*Don't shop hungry.* If you are hungry when you shop, you will buy more junk, quick snacks, processed foods, and fewer fruits and veggies.

*Buy in bulk,* but then put food into small bags or containers. We tend to finish whatever size we start.

*Make your home a safe zone.* Don't keep tempting junk food, bad snacks, processed food, cookies, or cake in the house. If you want something, make it from scratch with real ingredients. You will eat less because you won't make it as often.

## SHOP BY DESIGN

Shopping is a habit. You tend to habitually look for and buy the same few foods. The Daniel Plan launches you into a new mode of discovery, planning and rethinking how you shop for food. Once you learn what to look for and how to shop, how to "hunt and gather," how to learn what's available in the small radius where you live, then you can reclaim your health and vitality and live an abundant and full life.

A few key skills you need to shop well: (1) Learning to be an expert label reader; (2) finding the real food sources in your neighborhood; (3) learning how to navigate a supermarket, how to buy good food for less money, and how to use your grocery store as your "FARMacy."

## WHERE TO SHOP

Most Americans spend less than about 6 percent of their income on food, while Europeans spend 9 to 13 percent.[21] Rethinking your budget to include higher quality food is something that will pay off much greater dividends in energy, long-term health, and lower health care and prescriptions costs when you get older. You can pay a little more now or pay a lot more later. What is the real long-term cost of that French fry or soda for your health, your family, your neighborhood, and even the environment?

You will have to venture into new stores or into new places in your supermarket.

*Farmer's markets:* More and more communities have farmer's markets. They are a great place to see the face that feeds you and to find much more nutrient-dense, better-tasting food. Vegetables are no more expensive there than in most supermarkets and are often local, organic, and fresh and include unusual and funny varieties that pack more phytonutrients and taste. Fruit can be more expensive there, but once you try a fresh strawberry or peach from a farmer's market, you may never want to eat the store version again. Local and sustainably raised meats and organic cheeses and eggs are often available at farmer's markets. Find the one near you. Check out *localharvest.org* to find a market near you.

*Community-supported agriculture (CSA):* In most communities now, you can buy a "subscription" for the season to a local farm. Every week or month, depending on what you choose, you can pick up or have dropped off at your house a box of local, delicious organic fruits and vegetables for a fraction of the cost. Some CSAs also have eggs or sustainably raised meat or chicken. For cold climates, the season is shorter, but it is a fabulous way to eat well for less. You don't get to pick the food items, so view it as a great food adventure that will help you experiment with new vegetables and fruit. Check out *localharvest.org* to find and sign up for one in your community.

*Produce markets and ethnic grocers:* Look for produce markets or ethnic grocers in your neighborhood. Asian markets often have wonderful vegetables, including unusual varieties.

*Food co-ops:* These are found in communities and provide good, fresh, local food. You can buy items in bulk such as whole grains, beans, nuts, and seeds.

*Supermarkets:* The key here is to shop around the perimeter of the store. That is where you will find the produce, meat, fish, eggs, and dairy. It is not danger-free, but it is where you should spend most of your time. The aisles are "danger zones," so try to find anything that doesn't contain sugar, salt, or trans fats. You will be hunting a long time. Sometimes you need to venture down the aisles to find the beans, nuts, whole grains, salsa, hot sauce, olive oil, vinegar, condiments, and spices. Visit The Daniel Plan website for "Supermarket Savvy — The Good Stuff" and "Supermarket Savvy — The Bad Stuff."

### Grocery Shopping Tip

The ends of the aisles display the worst foods, such as 2-liter sodas, giant sugared cereal boxes, and worse. In the aisles, the worst food items are at eye level; the better-for-you foods are often on the bottom or top shelves.

*Big ticket stores:* Wal-Mart, Costco, Sam's Club, BJ's Wholesale, and Trader Joe's all have great buys at good prices. Explore yours. They increasingly have organic foods. You must be careful not to buy more than you need. It is a great way to stock up on organic olive oil, nuts, sardines, and even fruits and vegetables. Being a smart shopper in these stores can help you feed your family well for less.

*Convenience stores:* The only safe thing to buy at these stores is water, toilet paper, and fresh fruit, which many of these stores have started to carry.

## HOW TO READ LABELS

Becoming an expert label reader is your most essential shopping skill. There are two parts of the label: the nutrition facts, which are not that helpful; and the ingredient list, which is what you need to study.

The main thing to know about the nutrition facts is the total calories and serving size. A bag of whole grain baked chips may say 4 servings, but who shares? The calorie count is per serving, so multiply the serving size by calorie count to get the true amount you are eating. Look for total carbohydrates and carbohydrates from sugar. It should have less than 10 grams or consider it dessert. More than 5 grams of fiber is good, and more than 10 grams of protein is also good.

The real place to look for what you are actually eating is on the ingredient list. The good news is that more and more manufacturers are packaging real, whole food that is convenient *and* good to eat. If you follow these simple rules, you will stay out of trouble:

*Choose only real food.* If there are any words on the label that you don't recognize or can't pronounce, are in Latin, or sound like some science project, then put it back on the shelf. A jar of tomatoes, a can of artichokes, a curry sauce, a bottle of balsamic vinegar — they are examples of real food.

*Think five or less.* If it is a real food product, it usually has less than five ingredients. Some newer, healthier products contain more, but they are all real food.

***Don't buy anything with the three most dangerous ingredients.*** (You have them memorized by now, don't you?)

***Watch out for health claims.*** Anything with a health claim is almost guaranteed to be bad for you — diet this or low-fat that or trans fat free or low calorie or cholesterol lowering.

*Be alert to pseudonyms for sugar.* There are more than 250 names for hidden sugar in our food supply. Often packaged foods will contain four to six (or more) forms of sugar. Read carefully.

What comes first? Ingredients are listed in order of quantity. If you see sugar or salt as the first or second ingredient, then it's probably not a good idea to eat it. If it has more than 15 grams of sugar, it has more sugar than a glazed donut.

Visit The Daniel Plan website (*danielplan.com*) for more guidance on understanding labels.

## Health Food Imposters

- Sweetened yogurt has more sugar than the average soda.
- Watch the soy. Most processed GMO soy foods are harmful, not healthy. Traditional soy products such as tofu, tempeh, and miso are fine.
- Meat alternatives or fake meat such as hot dogs or burgers often contain gluten, processed soy, and bad oils.
- Protein bars often contain trans fat, high fructose corn syrup or sugar substitutes, and a load of weird ingredients.
- Eat only whole food bars made from nuts, seeds, and fruits.
- Fruit juice is liquid sugar — a treat, not a health food.

## HEALTHY EATING ON A BUDGET

Making real food from scratch from real ingredients is cheaper and tastier than outsourcing our food making to the industrial food system. In terms of cost per nutrient, processed foods are infinitely more expensive. We often crave more food because we are nutrient deficient.

> Eating nutrient dense food will naturally cut our cravings and our appetite and lead to deeper satisfaction with food and eating.

You have to be smart about your choices. There are valuable resources for those who want to find better food at a lower cost. The Environmental Working Group (*ewg.org*) created a wonderful guide called *Good Food on a Tight Budget*. Here are a few ideas that can save you money and save your health.

*Buy things in season.* Getting foods in season will always be cheaper. Buy strawberries in June, not January, when they have to be shipped from Mexico.

*Get frozen fruits and veggies.* When foods are not in season, frozen is the next best thing.

*Eat beans and whole grains.* These are good foods that feed most of the world for less than a dollar a day. Include more of them in your diet.

*Cook in bulk.* Make stews and soups, and store extra beans and grains. They store well in the fridge for three to four days.

*Freeze it.* If you make extra food, you can freeze it for later. Soups and stews are great for this.

*Stock up on staples.* When things such as olive oil, vinegars, and frozen foods are on sale, get them.

*Buy bigger sizes.* Divide what you buy into smaller containers and store or freeze.

*Cut it up.* Buy fruits and veggies you can cut up and store in containers in the fridge ready to eat. You will tend to eat what is easy, so taking a few minutes for slicing, peeling, and storing will help you make cheaper, healthier choices when you want a snack.

*Go green.* Eating big bunches of greens is a cheap way to get a filling, power-packed meal. We recommend eating 2 cups a day of some types of greens — salad mix, arugula, spinach, kale, collards, dandelion greens, and escarole.

*Make soup.* When veggies start to get a little old in the fridge, it is time to make soup. A few beans, some spices, and a good recipe can turn questionable vegetables into an unquestionably good meal.

*Stock up on long-lasting veggies,* including carrots, fingerling or small red potatoes, sweet potatoes, winter squash, onions, celery, and cabbage.

*Get protein for less.* Get good local or low-mercury small frozen fish or shrimp from big-ticket stores. Buy a whole chicken or turkey, roast it, and eat it over a few days.

*Get nut butters in bulk,* which you can find at food co-ops.

## COOKING BY DESIGN

"I first learned about food from my mother," Dr. Hyman says. "I want to celebrate my mother because she taught me something so essential and enduring that it has become my greatest passion: food and cooking. And through cooking, touching, feeling, preparing, and savoring good, real food made from real ingredients, I get to fully inhabit my kitchen; heal my body; and connect with friends, family, the Earth, and the larger community in which I live."

Mothers are exactly the allies we need to lead this food and cooking revolution. Cooking is a transformational act. The closer we can get to the food we eat, the shorter the link between field and fork, the better off we will all be. We have outsourced our cooking to the industrial food system. By taking back our kitchens — which we can do simply, easily, and inexpensively — we can create a tidal shift in our food system, homes, and communities.

### Who Knew?

The Kluge family grew up in homes where things were either fried or eaten out of a box or can. They made only two vegetables: boiled cabbage and canned green beans. They didn't have basic cooking implements, such as proper cutting boards to cut vegetables or even meat. They had some old, dull knives they never used hidden under the cupboard. Tinna, the mom, didn't know how to chop a vegetable or sauté it. They spent about $1,000 a month on food, half of it eating out in fast-food places.

So when Dr. Hyman visited the Kluge family, he realized the best way he could help them was not to prescribe medication or tell them to eat less and exercise more, but to teach them to cook real food from scratch. He got the whole family cooking,

"My mother was given the gift of knowing food through her mother, which she then gifted to me, helping me learn the beautiful connections between gardening, cooking, eating, and wellness," Dr. Hyman says. "And I have taught that to my children who have become wildly gifted cooks — making delicious home-cooked meals from real ingredients."

The most important food skill you have to create a rich, abundant, healthy life is this: *cooking*. Cooking at home can be faster and cheaper than eating out. Cooking a meal at home with family or friends, sharing the meal, and celebrating life and food together is one of life's greatest pleasures.

Cooking is one of those acts that we have been doing for thousands of years. Ritual, tradition, and connection around food are part of every culture. In the time it takes to cook most packaged foods, you can make yourself a simple, delicious, healthy meal from real ingredients. You just have to have them in the house ready to go.

washing, peeling, chopping, cutting, and touching real food. He showed them how to peel garlic, cut onions, and snap asparagus to get rid of the chewy parts. He taught Tinna how to sauté them in olive oil and garlic, to roast sweet potatoes with fennel and olive oil, and to make turkey chili from scratch. They even made fresh salad dressing from olive oil, vinegar, mustard, and salt and pepper.

After a happy, filling, healing meal of real food, one of the teens said in disbelief, "Dr. Hyman, do you eat real food like this with your family every night?"

Five days after Dr. Hyman's visit, Tinna texted Dr. Hyman that her family had already lost 18 pounds, and she was making his chili from scratch. After three months, Tinna lost 47 pounds, and her husband and son both lost 30 pounds — from cooking their own meals at home from scratch.

To succeed in the kitchen:

*Get the right equipment.* A few sharp knives will last a lifetime and make easy work of chopping and cutting vegetables. Good pans are easier to use and create better results.

*Learn basic cooking skills.* You can take a class, but today you can learn almost any basic cooking skill online.

*Start with knife skills.* YouTube is a great place to start.

*Plan ahead.* Set time aside for shopping every week. Plan your meals, and make your grocery list. Ideally you can shop just once a week if you plan your weekly meals and snacks. We are all busy, but shopping for real food is the best hour or two you will spend every week.

*Prepare well.* If you can read, you can cook! Getting all the ingredients out, even measured, before you start to cook makes quick work of any meal. Read the recipe carefully. Check out *danielplan.com* for new recipe ideas.

*Know when it's done.* The hardest part of cooking is learning when something is done. The vegetables should still be crisp, not soggy and limp. Overcooked chicken, meat, or fish is chewy and tough. You want to cook it until the pink is just gone. Fish is ready when it starts to flake apart when touched. Red meats should be cooked medium rare or medium.

If you are new to cooking from scratch, *start with simple meals.* Use just a few ingredients. Once you find a few quick simple dinners or lunches that you and your family like, keep the ingredients in your fridge or freezer so you are never stuck. Use the forty-day core meal plan in chapter 10 to get started.

Another thing is to *make the kitchen fun.* Put on great music, listen to podcasts of your favorite show, and invite family members and friends to share the preparation and cooking. If you have fun in the kitchen, you won't be afraid to get in there and cook more often.

Take baby steps, start simply, and realize that in very short order you can become comfortable in the kitchen and prepare quick, inexpensive, delicious meals to feed yourself and your family.

system. Aligning what we eat with who we are and our core values will make it much easier to change our habits. That is why all five Essentials are so tightly connected.

The solution is actually in each one of our hands. Literally. It is the power of your fork! What you choose to put on your fork is a powerful influence to change our individual health, food production practices, food policies, health care costs, and the health of the environment. By making simple changes in your food choices and cooking real food made from real ingredients, you will not only restore your health and your family's health, but can also contribute to changing what is wrong with our food and health care system.

The Daniel Plan is about taking back your health. But it is also about the health of your family, your church, your community, and your world. That is why we believe that once The Daniel Plan is embraced by the faith community, it will spread the gospel of health and change through America and the world.

### Reflect and Take a Step ...

So your goal is to eat real, whole food. Food that grows on a plant versus processed foods that do your body harm. It's all about learning to love foods that love you back. Make it your goal to follow The Daniel Plan plate 90 percent of the time. And always remember: It's about progress, not perfection.

## GROW YOUR OWN

While not everyone can grow their own food, most of us can d(
thing to include fresh, local food in our lives. Have a pot of he
your windowsill. Put a few simple plants such as cherry tomat(
peppers in a pot in your backyard or on the deck. Raised bed ga₁
ing is easy and can be done in a small area. Urban rooftop agricul
is an emerging trend.

While you may not want to become an organic farmer, growin₁
few things that you can watch grow, tend, and eat will connect you
real, fresh food in a way nothing else can. It is the best way to get kic
excited about eating vegetables. Start small, get help from someon(
who has done it, get a book, watch a few online videos, or join a local
community garden where you can share in the work and rewards. The
Daniel Plan website offers several cooking demonstration videos.

## TAKING BACK YOUR HEALTH —
## AND THE WORLD'S

There are personal reasons to do The Daniel Plan: to feel better, to
lose weight, to support those in your family or faith community. Food
is a personal issue tied to our culture, habits, and preferences. But the
implications of what we eat are much greater. How does what we eat
connect to our values and purpose in life? How do the choices we
make affect our family, our neighborhood, and our society?

When a twelve-year-old needs a liver transplant from drinking too
much soda, it's an indication that our food choices have moved beyond
the realm of individual personal responsibility. Faith-based communities have been among the first to act when human rights are violated.
No one wants to see our human communities eroded by disease and
disability. No one wants to see us destroy our own backyards and the
very land that sustains us. The erosion of our health has become a
social justice issue, a human rights issue. The right to health is among
the most basic of human rights.

Individuals and their communities, social networks, and connections have tremendous power to change everything about our food

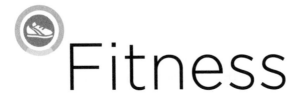

# Chapter 5

# Fitness

*Do you not know that your bodies are temples of the Holy
  Spirit…?*
*Therefore honor God with your bodies.*
*(1 Corinthians 6:19 – 20)*

Doreen was a middle-aged single mother of two boys with a lot on her plate and mind. When she walked into the fitness facility that exercise physiologist Foy trained in, he noticed she looked tired and had sad eyes. She mustered up a brave smile and said:

> "Do you think you can help me? I've tried a lot of different ways to improve my health, but exercise has not really been high on my list. My doctor told me I needed to start exercising right away. I am not sure I'm going to like it, and I'm afraid I won't be very good at it."

You see, Doreen wanted to find a way to lose an unwanted extra 30 pounds that had slowly accumulated over the years of raising a family and working full time. She also wanted to lower her dangerously high blood pressure and cholesterol and recapture her vitality. As she told Foy, "I'd really like to get that 'spark' back to my life!" He asked some questions to understand what made Doreen tick, and he walked her through these steps that make fitness doable in The Daniel

> Make fitness doable: Dream big, discover what moves you, set and record goals, mix it up, and find a buddy.

Plan: dreaming big, discovering what moves you, setting and recording goals, mixing it up, and finding a buddy.

Doreen is now 30 pounds lighter, in amazing physical shape, has blood pressure and cholesterol levels of a healthy 20-year-old — and by the way, she is now in her mid-eighties! She loves to exercise every day and is younger physically today than she was when she was in her forties. How do we know this? Doreen is Foy's mother! The best part is that she got her "spark" back.

Foy's mom became what we call Daniel Strong. Not only is she physically healthy, but she is also emotionally, relationally, and spiritually fit and pursues excellence in all she does for God's glory. Like the prophet Daniel, she is an example of faith, devotion, dedication, discipline, love, joy, and fearlessness.

## DANIEL STRONG

What images come to mind when you think of the word *strong*? A powerful 300-pound football player? An Olympic Gold medalist weightlifter? Do you think of the prophet Daniel? Daniel possessed strength that went well beyond the size of his muscles. He had a strength of faith, courage, obedience, devotion, dedication, endurance, and discipline in body, mind, and spirit. That is where we get the concept of Daniel Strong.

DANIEL STRONG  =  *A pursuit of excellence in body, mind, and spirit for God's glory.*

Daniel demonstrated his pursuit of excellence in his faithfulness in doing the little things when no one was watching. He had strength to do what was honoring to God, what was right, even in the face of danger or conflict or against what everyone else was doing. And that's exactly what is required to experience becoming Daniel Strong. There will be some days when you don't feel like pursuing excellence in your exercise, your eating, or your faith. But over time, pursuing excellence will lead to strength of character, confidence, and courage forged by God.

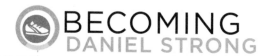

# BECOMING
## DANIEL STRONG

**IF YOU WERE TO ASK TEN PEOPLE** if they believe exercise is good for their health and well-being, how many of them do you think would raise their hands? If you guessed nine out of ten, you would match what we all intuitively know to be true. Exercise is good for us. But what do you think is the number one exercise that will help you look and feel younger, ramp up a sluggish metabolism, reduce and manage your weight, boost your energy, enhance creativity and productivity, increase cardiovascular endurance, improve muscular tone and strength, enhance sleep, reverse heart disease and high blood pressure and diabetes, reduce stress, and bring joy and youthfulness back to your life?

The number one exercise to help you attain all of these benefits … is the one you will do!

It's true. Despite all the research surrounding the benefits of regular exercise, the only one that will make a difference is the program you do consistently.

But we have a problem. Only about half of us exercise three or more days a week.[1] The amazing health and life-changing benefits of exercise we all know about don't motivate the majority of us to get off the sofa or easy chair and move.

Let's get to the bottom of this. What if you wanted to exercise? What if you were inspired and truly motivated to lace up your gym shoes and go for a walk, a run, or a hike? What if you moved from thinking, *I know I should exercise* to *I can't wait to exercise* and, by integrating motion with devotion, you could grow closer and stronger in your relationship with God? What if you discovered the moves that made you feel younger and recaptured the joy and fun of your youth?

## DESIGNED TO MOVE

For years now, researchers and health professionals have demonstrated that physical activity and exercise have a significant impact on our physical and mental health.[2] We were designed to move. In fact, God created each of us to move. Think about the countless activities you perform throughout your busy day — from getting out of bed to putting your clothes on, from driving to work to working all day, and [you name it].

The intricate body systems God put in place for the simplest of tasks, such as brushing our teeth or tying our shoes, are nothing short of miraculous. From the thought of *I need to brush my teeth,* which requires activating brain cells, to the nerves, muscles, ligaments, tendons, and bones all working together, the flow of movement occurs beautifully.

Whatever you find yourself doing throughout your day, it most likely demands you to move your body in some form or fashion to complete a given task — and none of this could be accomplished without your muscles. Muscles help us stand, sit, walk, bend, stretch, twist, push, pull, reach, and carry.

## SLOWING DOWN

For most of human history, our ancestors were constantly moving. They were hunters, gatherers, farmers, homemakers, soldiers, and more. Their lives consisted of much physical activity or physical labor throughout the day.

They didn't have to think about exercise, because their entire day required exercise. Their muscles and bodies were strong, fit, and productive. It wouldn't be uncommon for one of our ancestors to expend the caloric equivalent of walking ten miles in one day. Many a middle-aged man of years ago could pick up objects or sustain physical exertion levels that most eighteen-year-olds today would find extremely difficult. It wasn't until the later part of the eighteenth century, with the Industrial Revolution, that machines began to replace many of the daily movements and activities people were used to doing.

Fast-forward to today and we are now in the age of the computer, cell phone, remote, escalator, and elevator. Movement has been slowly removed from our daily living, and we are, unfortunately, reaping the costs with compromised health, excess weight, aches and pains, premature aging, and weak muscles. How can we reverse this trend and make our bodies young and strong again?

Do we have some great news for you! Truth be told, you can make exercise a reality and discover movement you truly enjoy. When exercise is a part of your life because you want it, enjoy it, and are inspired by it, you will reap its benefits immensely. We will teach you proven fitness tips and relate stories of real people who have discovered the life-changing benefits and joy of exercise.

## TAKE A PICTURE

Imagine that you have a digital camera in hand to take a picture of yourself. Now, don't be nervous, but take a "picture" of your current health and fitness. Give yourself plenty of grace, and don't be critical, but take an honest peek from head to toe.

- How is your energy level?
- How do you feel most days?
- How is your weight?
- What do you notice about your face, shoulders, arms, abs, and legs?
- How does your present fitness level impact your faith, food choices, focus, family, work, ministry — and life in general?

Once you have thought through these questions, is there anything about your current picture of health and fitness that concerns you?

Now imagine yourself five years older than you are today and in the best physical shape you have ever known. Picture yourself Daniel Strong — physically, emotionally, relationally, and spiritually fit. Go ahead and take a snapshot of your fitness and health five years from now.

We can only imagine what you would be able to do then. But

there would be activities you could enjoy that you can't today. Your thoughts, emotions, and experiences with and about your body would be much different.

## DREAM BIG!

"I have a dream!" Everyone knows those famous words that echoed through the crowds at the Lincoln Memorial in Washington, DC, on August 28, 1963. These simple, yet profound words by Dr. Martin Luther King Jr. sparked a great decline in racism in the United States and was the defining moment of the American Civil Rights Movement. What began as a dream and vision of what could be ultimately became a national movement, leading to freedom and justice for millions of Americans.

> Ask yourself, "If I could realize or accomplish anything related to my fitness and health, without fear of failure, what would it be?"

In many ways, dreaming is the first step to accomplishing almost any endeavor. It is no different with fitness. To get moving, we need to begin with your big dream.

To inspire you to dream big, here are a few dreams from others who have embarked on The Daniel Plan:

- Help build a school in India
- Complete a 5K run
- Learn to swim
- Do 100 push-ups without rest
- Hike through the Grand Canyon
- Compete in an Iron Man triathlon
- Scuba dive off the Barrier Reef
- Start a softball team
- Get a black belt in karate
- Cycle across the state with grandkids
- Compete in the next Olympic games
- Kayak through Alaska
- Climb the Great Wall of China
- Complete a marathon in every state

You may find it difficult to capture a big fitness dream right now, and that's okay. Before you set your big fitness dream, take some time to ask God to show you what you would love to do, be, or experience related to your fitness a few years from now.

## ONE WORD TO MOVE

Now take a moment to think about your main motivator to propel you toward your fitness dream and a lifetime of health. To help you through this process, we want you to think about your reason a little bit differently.

Dan Britton, Jimmy Page, and Jon Gordon, in their fascinating book entitled *One Word That Will Change Your Life,* present the idea of focusing on one word every year to help transform your life.[3] We can apply this wisdom to finding one word for the changes you want to make on The Daniel Plan. For example, if your dream is to run the Boston Marathon, your one-word reason may be *challenge* or *accomplishment.* Maybe your dream is to start a hiking club and tour different parts of the world, so your word might be *enjoyment* or *fellowship.*

The authors share three steps to help you identify your word, your one reason to begin to move more:

1. Look *in* to prepare your heart.
2. Look *up* to God to help you discover your one word.
3. Look *out* with the help of others to help you live your word.

What one word comes to mind for why you want to accomplish and long to achieve your particular fitness dream?

| | |
|---|---|
| ☐ Accomplishment | ☐ Fellowship |
| ☐ Adventure | ☐ Fun |
| ☐ Challenge | ☐ Joy |
| ☐ Enjoyment | ☐ Kids/Grandkids |
| ☐ Excitement | ☐ Service |
| ☐ Excellence | ☐ Spouse |
| ☐ Family | ☐ Youthfulness |
| ☐ Faith | ☐ Worship |

Feel free to add to the list and identify your one word. Following what you enjoy, and with the help of God and others, you will gain the motivation, encouragement, direction, and strength to help you become Daniel Strong.

---

**John's Word**

I was standing in the buffet line at our annual men's retreat behind one of our pastors. He turned to me and said, "Sean, I'd really like to lose 40 pounds. I know what you do for a living, and I'd like your help." Before I could say anything, he continued, "Let me tell you why I want to lose 40 pounds. Yes, it would be great to look and feel better and be able to do some of the things I used to do. But my real reason for losing weight and getting in shape is that I want to share and preach the gospel of Christ's love with as many people as I can. Before I [leave this life] I hope to share the gospel with thousands more. I'm in my sixties right now, and I want to be fit to serve God for as long as I possibly can."

John defined his dream, his greater purpose for getting and staying fit. What would his one word be? Service. He wanted to be Daniel Strong to serve God as long as he could. John got fit and lost weight, but more important, he is still ministering and serving today.

—Exercise Physiologist Sean Foy

---

## JUST ONE STEP

With the majority of our to-do lists and goals soon forgotten, how do we keep a dream alive and move forward?

Dreams — what we hope to accomplish — give birth to our goals, the steps we are willing to take to reach our dreams. Goals are the steps we take each day, week, and month to get from where we are today to the future we dream of having. Unfortunately, most of us

## It's a Date

"Trying to exercise on my own — I have a lot of excuses why I can't — but to have an appointment, a set day, that I go to Zumba has really been a plus.

"I'm one of the older ladies, and that's okay. It's a lot easier to exercise with other people and to be in a group of people who don't judge you if you do the exercises incorrectly. Most times I'm going to the left while everyone else is going to the right. That's okay. They can do splits. I just kind of bend my knees, and that's okay."

— Mary Clements

don't take the time to write down what we hope to attain, nor do we take the time to determine the steps to get us there, especially when it comes to our fitness.

Making fitness a part of our lives can be compared to planning a long trip. Some trips are well planned and can withstand any difficulty. Others are not, and we end up in the wrong destination. If you were planning a trip of a lifetime, such as hiking through the Grand Canyon, you would take time not only to plan your trip, but also to be in the best shape possible to enjoy it.

Likewise, to reach your health and fitness destination, it is important to begin mapping out a few markers or milestones along the way. If you don't like to set goals because you find the process too cumbersome, we want to assure you that there are different means of goal setting.

### OPTION 1: ONE WORD

Take the one word idea a little farther. Think about one word each week or month related to your fitness, and use that as your guiding light to help you pursue excellence. For example, let's say your word today or this week is *endurance*. With this one word, focus the majority of your energy and efforts on doing as many different forms of exercise that improve or enhance your endurance. The next week maybe your word is *strength*. This focus will propel you to look for ways to increase your strength for the week.

This "one word" focus is a great method to help you pursue excellence in different areas of your personal fitness.

Now, if you are someone who likes to set goals, I would encourage you to take a moment to answer the following questions to help map your course.

### OPTION 2: MAP YOUR FITNESS COURSE

Identify the benefits to accomplishing your fitness dream:

1. _____

2. _____

Identify the obstacles to achieving your fitness dream:

1. _____

2. _____

List your solutions to overcoming your obstacles:

1. _____

2. _____

Determine a date when you would like to accomplish your big dream.

Forty days from today, what would you like to realize or accomplish?

You can use *The Daniel Plan Journal* or App to set goals and record your journey to the destination. Now that you have determined your initial word or markers, we want to inspire you to find what moves you.

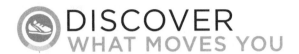

# DISCOVER
## WHAT MOVES YOU

**ON A WARM SUMMER NIGHT** Charles Whitley, a new resident of Sunnyvale rest home, strains and sighs as he carefully leans his eighty-two-year-old body forward to get a better look. Charles peers through his upstairs window, intently watching the neighborhood children play kick the can. Reminiscing, he searches his memories for days filled with running, jumping, skipping, hiding, and the familiar *ting* of a can and shouts of laughter.

One day Charles shares an idea with his old friend, Ben Conroy. He wonders aloud, "What if playing kick the can could somehow magically make us young again? Ben, did you ever stop to think of it? All kids play kick the can or hide and seek, and the minute they stop playing, they begin to grow old. It's almost as though playing kick the can keeps them young."

> "We do not quit playing because we grow old; we grow old because we quit playing."
> —Oliver Wendell Holmes

Late one night Ben watches in amazement as Charles leads a group of his elderly housemates onto the front lawn to play kick the can. As Ben rubs his eyes, he gasps at what he sees. One moment Charles and his feeble senior playmates are shuffling out the door, and the next they are magically transformed into their young ten-year-old carefree selves, skipping and running off into the warm summer night.

This tale, from the classic 1960s TV series *Twilight Zone*, makes you wonder if Charles Whitley was on to something.

Believe it or not, you can turn back the clock to some degree and re-energize your body, mind, and heart. We want to invite you to sneak away from old ways of thinking about fitness in order to learn from others who have successfully uncovered the secret to staying young, healthy, and fit.

## REMEMBER WHEN

Picture yourself when you were a fifth grader, probably ten or eleven years old. Do you remember ...

- Looking into the sky watching clouds morph into zoo animals and cartoon characters?
- Running with outstretched arms like Superman or Wonder Woman, saving the entire city?
- Playing tag, getting caught, and laughing so hard you couldn't breathe?
- Climbing trees?
- Running and jumping into a pile of leaves?
- Not worrying about how much you weighed, what you looked like, what clothes you wore, or how much money you had?
- Skipping, hiding, seeking, shooting, chasing, swimming, dancing, and catching?

When we were young, moving our bodies was a natural part of our day. We looked forward to recess. We longed for it. We dreamt about it. We waited patiently for the school bell to ring or our next-door neighbor to come home to play. We were always in motion.

## PLAY LIKE A KID

Dr. William Sears, "America's Pediatrician," is the father of eight children and a bestselling author and, most important, loves kids. He asked fitness expert Foy to coauthor a book with him and his son Peter, called *Lean Kids*.

With the desire to help children combat inactivity and obesity, they set out to create a proven program that would be implemented in schools, after-school facilities, churches, and community centers throughout the United States. They knew that to help kids move more, they would need to come up with a fun way of building activity back into their lives. They thought it would be easy.

What they didn't realize was how much activity had been removed from our children's lives. In performing their research, Dr. Sears and Foy looked at movement patterns of youth years ago. They also fondly remembered when they were young, playing outdoors. Today, for our kids, it is just the opposite. With tablets, smart phones, and online games, kids today need to be coaxed to go outside. They spend much of their days sitting down and therefore experience some of the same health and fitness challenges as adults three times their age.

So Foy and the Searses went to work, with a passion and desire to design a curriculum and program geared to help kids get moving again. They created the PLAY program and implemented it in

## The Difference a Ride Makes

"A few years ago I went on a hike with a friend and saw a group of ladies doing a mountain bike clinic. They invited us to join their group, and the next day I signed up online. I had no idea I would have so much fun riding a bike or how much my life would change because of this group activity. It's become like a sisterhood for me as I learned to take to the trails with people who support and cheer me on every time we ride.

"The leader of The Trail Angels inspires and often encourages us to get out of our comfort zones. With the confidence she has taught me on the bike, I'm now leading beginners on their first rides.

"Mountain biking has also become a kind of therapy for me. If I'm having a rough day, a quick mountain bike ride with friends changes my outlook and clears my head. Our rides are often filled with laughter. A crash or a flat tire often turns into an opportunity to take funny pictures to post on Facebook. Some rides have themes or costumes, and we've been known to do scavenger hunts while riding. This kind of fun with fitness is contagious. I'm always thinking about my next ride and wondering who I can invite to join me!"

— Tracy Jones

various after-school facilities. After the initial pilot programs, they were pleased to see that children improved not only their strength, flexibility, endurance, balance, coordination, weight loss, and overall fitness and health, but also their confidence, self-esteem, emotional well-being, relationships, and quality of life.[4]

Foy and the Searses knew they were onto something. Today there are more than 1,000 certified LEAN coaches who are helping kids and families get fit throughout the world. That same program is the basis for the PLAY concept of The Daniel Plan.

## BACK TO THE JOY OF PLAY

Back then we called it *play*, and we *loved* every minute of it. Today, for many, we call it *exercise* and *count* every minute of it, longing for it to be over. We frequently find it painful, boring, or dull, and we feel guilty about not doing it. For many of us, the results of tomorrow are just not worth the effort today. Many of us won't switch to an active lifestyle just because it's good for us. So what will change us?

Kay Warren said, "You were meant for something more. You were

### Sitting Disease

Believe it or not, the average American employee will sit anywhere from 7.7 to 15 hours a day without moving.[5] Researchers are now beginning to unravel the catastrophic impact that sitting for long periods of time can cause to human health. Experts have coined the phrase "sitting disease" to describe it. This is what the science is saying:

• The University of Missouri discovered that sitting for three to four hours at a time actually shuts off your body's ability to burn fat efficiently. Researchers discovered that a fat-burning enzyme called *lipoprotein lipase* loses its ability to be absorbed when you are seated for long periods of time.[6]

meant to experience a life of joy." God designed us to experience joy. In fact, we crave it and search for it. Unfortunately, when stress builds up, joy escapes us, and we wind up overeating, overworking, over-stressing, overdoing, and even over-sitting. Most of our days are spent with long spans of minimal movement, which impacts not only our joy, but also our bodies.

The Daniel Plan integrates motion with devotion and brings back the fun and joy to your fitness and life.

It makes sense, doesn't it? Sure, we can pop in the extreme fitness DVD or drag ourselves to the gym for a few weeks or months, but sooner or later, if we don't enjoy what we are doing, we are going to find a way out. Why spend time enduring workouts we don't enjoy when we can experience all the health and fitness benefits of a complete exercise program that gives us fun learning to PLAY again?

Prayerful movements throughout your day

Loosening breaks

Active games and aerobic activity

Youthful strength training

- According to the Mayo Clinic, sitting is now the new smoking! Sitting too long, up to three to four hours at a time, is now equivalent to smoking a pack-and-a-half of cigarettes a day.[7] Yikes!

- The *British Journal of Sports Medicine* determined that individuals who sit too long — again, longer than three to four hours — significantly increase their risk of disease. But they also found that people who move just a little bit — even fidgeting or getting up from their desks on a frequent basis to get a cup of coffee, or taking a flight of stairs — significantly improved their health.[8]

All of the elements found in the PLAY method are essential to an effective fitness program. Some of them are also designed to help strengthen your relationship to God. By applying this simple method to your day, you will recapture your strength and the joy of moving again.

## P — PRAYERFUL MOVEMENTS THROUGHOUT YOUR DAY

So here's the good news. To begin to improve your health and fitness, you don't have to get sweaty. You don't have to put on gym clothes. You don't have to lift weights or even get a gym membership. Begin to boost your metabolism, energy, creativity, fitness, and health by performing simple movements throughout your day. Research proves that performing movements such as standing or fidgeting or lightly stretching or (as you will learn) active games, aerobic activity, or strength training even for just a minute or two every hour through-out your day can make a big difference to your health and well-being — and combat sitting disease.[9] We suggest that you also use these movements to strengthen your relationship with God throughout your busy day.

Consider using an hourly reminder to move your body. Not only will you combat sitting disease and improve your health and fitness, but you can also connect with God through worship, thanksgiving, and prayer.

To help you experience motion and devotion throughout your busy day, here are a few ideas to help you from nine to five, or when-

"When movement is experienced as joy, it adorns our lives, makes our days go better, and gives us something to look forward to. When movement is joyful and meaningful, it may even inspire us to do things we never thought possible."

— Scott Kretchmar, Penn State University Professor of Exercise and Sports Science

ever you find yourself sitting for long periods of time. Set an alarm clock or your phone to remind you every hour to do two or three of the following:

- Stand up for 1 to 2 minutes, and thank God for the many blessings in your day and life. (Chapter 6 will inspire you even more with the power of gratitude for your mental health.)

- Stretch your shoulders and arms, but close your eyes to worship God in silence.

- Squat up and down 5 to 10 times while thinking about how you are becoming Daniel Strong. With each repetition, thank God for a strong, healthy body and the ability to move.

- Stretch your lower back and legs by slowly reaching down to touch your toes. Hold for a few seconds, stand, and repeat again for a minute, and let this be a posture that expresses your devotion to God as you humble yourself, bowing down to God's will in your life.

- Perform deep breathing for a couple of minutes. Inhale God's strength and goodness. Exhale any worry or concern you may be carrying, releasing it to him with each breath.

- Stand or pace when you are talking on the phone. With each step, think about how Daniel listened, walked, and talked with God throughout his day.

- Do 10 desk push-ups. Thank God for the use of your muscles and the health of your body.

- Go for a walking meeting instead of sitting in a conference room. Use this as a time of fellowship with others at work, like Daniel and his three faithful friends.

- Turn on some music and dance for a few minutes to your favorite song or worship music.

- Take a 2-minute recess. Use a hula hoop, jump rope, or Frisbee at work. Remind yourself that God loves when you smile and laugh and bring a cheerful and joyful heart to others. Your smile and laughter may be the one thing that brightens another's day.

> ### Cool Tip
>
> How would you like to rev up your metabolism, burn up to 200 – 300 extra calories a day, and get in shape without sweating much from 9 to 5? Go to danielplan.com for tips on setting hourly two-minute breaks throughout your day to move your body. You will love it!

- Take the stairs instead of the elevator. Use the time walking up the stairs to thank God for all he has done in your life. On the way down, share your concerns, anxieties, and worries with God.
- Stand when doing desk work. Every hour stand for 2 minutes, and let this be a reminder to you to stand for God in all you do. Daniel risked being arrested for praying. Let your standing, instead of sitting, strengthen you, not only physically, but also spiritually.

Can you imagine the impact performing simple movements such as these, along with regular prayer, will have on your life?

## L — LOOSENING BREAKS

Research from the American Council on Exercise, the Mayo Clinic, the American College of Sports Medicine, and other established health and fitness organizations have determined that regular loosening, or stretching, activities performed throughout your day or before or after your workout can have a significant impact on your health, fitness, flexibility, and performance.[10] Take a look at just a few of the benefits loosening movements or activities can offer you:

- Decreases muscle stiffness, increases range of motion, and slows the physiological aging process of your joints

- Warms up your body and reduces risk of injury
- Helps relieve post-exercise aches and pains
- Improves posture and body symmetry
- Helps reduce or manage your stress
- Increases blood circulation, reduces muscular tension, and enhances muscular relaxation
- Improves your body's overall functional performance
- Prepares the body for the stress of exercise
- Promotes circulation and prevents injury
- Decreases the risk of lower back pain[11]

### Reduced Pain

"I played football at the University of Southern California in the early 1970s. From that alone, I had lower back pain and suffered from that greatly all the time. I had gone to a number of the high-level orthopedic surgeons, chiropractors, and acupuncturists — you pretty much name it. I wanted to be able to pick up my grandkids and hold them without dropping them because of the pain. Plus, my family was tired of me complaining. So when I heard about a stretching class [for one hour], I was the first guy to sign up. I had nothing to lose.

"There's nothing radical about it; it's very easy going. But after that hour of pure stretching, I'm a new guy. Now I not only can see my toes, but can actually touch them."

— Jim Lucas

Loosening movements or activities can be performed in two formats: statically or dynamically. Both increase flexibility of joints without stiffness or injury. This is important because flexible muscles, tendons, and ligaments can be less prone to soreness and injury and can help improve muscular performance. Think of your muscles as rubber bands. If you take a rubber band and quickly and forcefully stretch it past the point that it was intended to, the band will break. But by stretching it a little at a time and more each time, you can stretch it out farther and farther. By performing regular loosening breaks, you can increase the pliability of your joints to prevent "breaking," or injury.

Dynamic loosening, stretching as you are moving, prior to your exercise is the best way to warm up your body. Static loosening movements after you exercise is one of the best ways to enhance flexibility as well as minimize post-exercise aches and pains. But you can also perform loosening breaks throughout your day for fifteen to thirty seconds anywhere, anytime:

### STANDING ARM CIRCLES

1. Stand upright, with your feet hip-width apart, knees slightly bent, and your arms extended out to your sides, raised to shoulder level with your palms facing the floor.

2. Next, begin to make small, forward circular motions (about one foot in diameter) with your hands and arms in a controlled and slow fashion. Perform ten times.

3. Now, begin to increase the size of your shoulder arm circles by progressing to medium and then to larger circular motions, until you are reaching as far forward and back as you comfortably can (e.g., above your head and below your hips). Perform ten times.

4. Repeat the motion by following steps 2 and 3, but in reverse.

5. Perform ten times or for 15 to 20 seconds in each direction.

### TOE TOUCHES

1. Stand upright, with your feet tight together, legs straight, and your hands on your thighs (palms down).

2. Slowly and under control, bend forward at your waist (not your back), reaching down with your hands trying to touch your shins or toes.

3. Hold the stretch for 10 to 30 seconds.

*Note:* Warm up your muscles before performing this or any static stretch move. Also, if you have lower back problems, do not try toe touches like this. Instead, you may want to try a seated chair toe touch.

*Alternative:* Seated in a chair, with one leg extended, reach forward with both hands, bending from the waist, trying to reach your shins or toes.

If you have the time, you can participate in a class and enjoy loosening up for a full hour or more. To add extra loosening breaks to your day and exercise routine, choose from a few activities and resources:

- ☐ Ballet
- ☐ Gymnastics — try doing a somersault in your office if you want a laugh!
- ☐ Pilates or Pilates reformer
- ☐ Martial arts
- ☐ Massage
- ☐ Stability ball stretching
- ☐ Self-massage using a foam roller, ball, or stick
- ☐ Stretching with a towel or resistance bands
- ☐ Stretching at your desk at work

*Remember:* You can perform loosening breaks together or apart and as often as you would like throughout your day, even multiple times a day, every day of the week. You can also add prayer to use these breaks as your prayerful movement during your workday. Usually, loosening breaks should be anywhere from one to five minutes.

## A — ACTIVE GAMES AND AEROBIC ACTIVITY

What does *young at heart* mean to you? The *Chicago Tribune* was curious and asked its readers what they thought. Below are a few of the interesting answers they received:

**Rudolph Alfano, 80:** "To think young and be positive each and every single day. That's why I think I'm 16 years old because

I act like a kid sometimes. I stay young at heart by getting up early in the morning and going on my walk, going to bed early, eating fresh fruits and vegetables daily, working on a project each day, and helping others."

**William Danford, 91:** "It means having a wonderful nature that is attractive at all times."

**Lisa Dekter, 76:** "You realize that age is insignificant. To be 'young at heart' is to love life, wake up every day, and enjoy that day as a gift."[12]

Whatever your answer may be to this question, being "young at heart" is an endearing expression we use for people who enjoy doing things younger people like to do. We want to help you explore how to strengthen your heart as well as becoming young at heart by enjoying active games and aerobic activities.

## MORE THAN JUST A GAME

Active games and aerobic activity are beneficial to not only your physical heart, but also your social, mental, and spiritual heart. Playing outdoor or indoor games such as tag, jumping rope, or dodge ball are just a few examples of the many ways we used to play. Now you can begin to play again and reap the benefits.

Overwhelming scientific evidence supports the growing number of positive benefits for your body and health by performing active games and/or aerobic activity:

- Increasing lung capacity, muscle tone, and blood flow
- Stimulating your brain, sharpening listening skills, improving problem-solving skills
- Delaying age-associated memory loss
- Creating social ties and friendships
- Reducing risk of diabetes and high cholesterol
- Lowering risk of heart disease, cancer, and osteoporosis
- Strengthening the immune system

- Lowering levels of depression, stress, and anxiety
- Increasing self-esteem and self-image
- Managing stress
- Increasing ability to burn fat for energy
- Sleeping better
- Producing more energy
- Increasing productivity

*Bottom line:* Active games and aerobic exercise help your heart, lungs, and body stay fit and healthy, empowering you to be young at heart. The good news is, since your heart is a muscle, anything that challenges it — whether it's playing hopscotch, going for a hike, or walking up a flight of stairs — can strengthen it.

Researchers such as Dr. Stuart Brown, the founder of the National Institute for Play, classify play into different types or personalities.[13] Other researchers describe how our play personalities may be the

### Fit to Play

Tim Pidcock hadn't exercised consistently or seriously for decades after getting out of the military. Eventually his weight and health offered plenty of motivation to get fit, but one of his ongoing motivations was family vacation.

"We would be going for three weeks to Cebu, Philippines, where my wife is from. We had some fun activities planned, including river climbing, canyoning in Moalboal, and swimming with the whale sharks in Oslob. I wanted to be as fit as possible so I could enjoy these activities and more with my wife and kids without becoming a wheezing boat anchor. Our vacation was wonderful, and while the canyoning adventure was rained out, we had a great time river climbing and swimming with the whale sharks."

same as they were when we were kids or they may have changed over time. What about you? What type of play personality did you have when you were young? What about now? Fun, competition, challenge, education, or companionship can all be reasons to play.

When we think about aerobic exercise, we frequently think of things such as brisk walking, elliptical or stair climber machines, step classes, aqua aerobic classes, running, or interval training — which are all beneficial and will improve your health and fitness. But what about other activities we haven't played in a while that may bring that youthfulness and enjoyment back — games such as tennis, tag, handball, racquetball, and dodge ball?

Instead of dreading a "workout," add active games or aerobic activities to your day. Here are a few activities you can choose from that will help you be young at heart:

| | |
|---|---|
| ☐ Acrobatics | ☐ Racquetball |
| ☐ Badminton | ☐ Roller or ice skating/ |
| ☐ Backpacking |    roller blading |
| ☐ Baseball/softball | ☐ Rowing |
| ☐ Basketball | ☐ Skateboarding |
| ☐ Bowling | ☐ Skiing/snowboarding |
| ☐ Bicycling (stationary or road) | ☐ Soccer |
| ☐ Cross-country skiing | ☐ Snowshoeing |
| ☐ Dancing | ☐ Surfing |
| ☐ Dodge ball | ☐ Swimming |
| ☐ Fencing | ☐ Table tennis |
| ☐ Flag football | ☐ Tag |
| ☐ Frisbee golf | ☐ Tennis |
| ☐ Handball | ☐ Trampoline jumping |
| ☐ Horseback riding | ☐ Unicycling |
| ☐ Hula hooping | ☐ Ultimate Frisbee |
| ☐ Jumping rope | ☐ Volleyball |
| ☐ Mountain climbing | ☐ Wii Fit |
| ☐ Pogo stick | ☐ Zumba |

You can perform active games or aerobic activities every day of the week, but we recommend at least three to five days per week for twenty to sixty minutes. (If you don't have twenty minutes, even performing one to two or even ten minutes of cardio can be beneficial.) Also, mix it up or cross-train, which is performing different types of activity on varying days of the week, such as walking on Monday, rope jumping on Tuesday, cycling on Thursday, and going for a hike on Saturday. (See page 180 for more information on cross-training).

To improve your aerobic fitness and to help you become young at heart, challenge your body by increasing your heart rate during your selected activities. Your heart is a muscle, so when it is challenged, it will adapt and become stronger. Here is a good rule of thumb: When performing an aerobic activity or active game, you should find it challenging to carry on a lengthy conversation and feel winded, but you should be able to talk in short three-word sentences. If you can't converse at all, you are going too fast or hard. If you can sing comfortably during the activity, you are going too slow.

## Y — YOUTHFUL STRENGTH TRAINING

One of the most critical steps to recapturing our youth, vitality, and health is youthful strength training. Many of us think strength training is only for athletes. But you don't have to be an athlete to appreciate the benefits strength training can have on your body, mind, and life. Those who perform strength training on a regular basis, with a smile on their face, will be the first to tell you their body and mind feel years younger. Not to mention they are reaping a number of the other benefits. Be inspired by some of the benefits a youthful strength training program has on overall health and fitness:

- Boosts metabolism
- Manages weight and reduces body fat
- Improves posture
- Tones and firms muscles
- Improves mobility and balance

- Helps prevent osteoporosis
- Reduces stress and anxiety
- Decreases risk of injury
- Lowers risk of heart disease, cancer, blood pressure, diabetes, and arthritis (all of which can be pretty much resisted with healthy eating choices)
- Improves sleep

While these are all wonderful benefits and reasons to start "pumping" weights, we would like you to take a PLAY approach and identify the youthful strength training movement, activity, or class you would most enjoy. Ask yourself, "What would bring a smile to my face?"

- ☐ Barbell training
- ☐ Boot camp training
- ☐ Body calisthenics
- ☐ Canoeing/kayaking
- ☐ Circuit training
- ☐ CrossFit
- ☐ Dumbbell training
- ☐ Gymnastics
- ☐ Heavy rope lifting or swinging
- ☐ Kettlebell training
- ☐ Medicine ball training
- ☐ Pull-up bars
- ☐ Resistance bands
- ☐ Rock climbing
- ☐ Rowing machines
- ☐ Sand bag lifting, dragging, or throwing
- ☐ Sled training
- ☐ Strength training DVDs
- ☐ Suspension training (such as TRX, FKPro, or Aerosling)
- ☐ Tire flipping

To improve or maintain your muscular strength and endurance, it would be good to get to a place when your youthful strength training should consist of upper and lower body movements, using anywhere from five to ten different exercises, each with eight to fifteen repetitions. Perform one to three sets (a group of repetitions) at a moderate intensity for a minimum of two or three days a week.

Remember, if you only have time for one or two strength training movements, you will still find a number of benefits. You can perform youthful strength training exercises using just your body weight as part of your prayerful movements throughout your day and still see good results.

For example, you could perform the following movements several times each day:

☐ Ten squats          ☐ Ten dips          ☐ Ten lunges

(See chapter 9 for details on performing these movements correctly.)

Can you imagine how fit you would become performing this thirty-repetition routine even four times during your workday on a regular basis? By our count, you would have completed 120 repetitions for the day. Wow! You can get fit doing that! And if you add prayer during these short one-to-two-minute movements, imagine how it will improve your day and bring you closer to God.

Now, if you decide to do strength training using free weights or weight machines or in a challenging routine such as a boot camp or CrossFit with added weights or resistance, it is best to only do this routine every other day or two to three days per week. Give your body 24 to 48 hours to properly recover after a challenging strength workout. The best way to improve your fitness, strength, and/or muscular endurance is to challenge your muscles by progressing your intensity (number of reps, sets, or resistance) as you get stronger.

> "No discipline is enjoyable while it is happening—it's painful! But afterward there will be a peaceful harvest of right living for those who are trained in this way" (Hebrews 12:11 NLT).

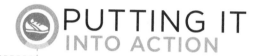

# PUTTING IT
## INTO ACTION

**NOW IT'S YOUR TURN.** Take the Daniel Strong Challenge to improve your fitness, combining prayerful movements, loosening breaks, active games and aerobic activity, and youthful strength training into your life, and watch what happens! We encourage you to do the fitness challenge for forty days to change your fitness habits. To begin — even if you have never exercised regularly or haven't in a long time — go to chapter 9, where you will receive a "play of the day" and a plan that focuses on all the aspects of fitness you have just learned — in small, doable steps.

To help you make consistent daily, weekly, and monthly progress to reach your goals and big fitness dream, monitoring and/or tracking your efforts is essential. In fact, in multiple studies, individuals who monitored their exercise habits significantly improved their behavior and likelihood of accomplishing their goals (just like the success with tracking your food choices). So how do you monitor your fitness?

1. Plan before your week begins.
2. Track your progress as well as the challenges.

## PLAN YOUR WEEK

Have you ever noticed that when you write something down with the intention of doing it, you usually do it? We have! Especially when it's important, such as lunch with a spouse or a close friend, attending our kids' events, or an important business meeting. There is something powerful in recording our plans and then checking them off as we successfully complete them. With each check, we gain confidence to make things happen and move closer to our long-term goals.

Imagine on Sunday evening, before your week begins, you were to sit down and pull out your smart phone or calendar and create a written "agreement" with yourself in which on Monday, Wednesday, and Friday from 6:30 p.m. to 7:30 p.m. you commit to your fitness, such as walking. Just typing it in instead of "hoping" to "get it in whenever you get a chance" increases your odds of completion. Think of it as a very important appointment.

### Full-Day Benefits

When it comes to exercise, researchers have found those who exercise in the morning are much more likely to eat healthier, exercise more, and take better care of themselves throughout the day.[14]

Sit down the night before or on a Sunday and determine your PLAY activities for the next day. Or if you prefer to be more spontaneous, make a list of PLAY activities you enjoy and each day select what you feel like doing.

Every Sunday evening Sean Foy sits down with his phone calendar and schedules his PLAY for the week. Many of his clients follow the same ritual. These are nonnegotiable appointments that Foy makes with either his fitness buddies or himself. If someone asks him for a meeting during that time, he typically will tell them that he has an appointment. Usually they respond, "No problem, how about a different time?"

By intentionally planning for the week before it happens, you create margin or space in your busy week and prioritize your efforts before things get crazy.

**Set realistic goals.** It's always best to set goals that you are confident you can accomplish. We encourage you to dream big, but it is important not to set fitness goals that are unrealistic. Remember, you don't have to be an elite athlete to be fit — just moving more than you did yesterday is a great step in the right direction.

## Couch to CrossFit

"This whole thing [starting The Daniel Plan] started when my sister Emily told me about a boot camp class. I was a little nervous about it, because I really had never done an exercise class before but thought I would give it a try—and let me tell you, it nearly killed me the first few times.

"Over the last year, I have had such a blast with the exercise programs offered at Saddleback Church. At the beginning, I was 280 pounds and would get out of breath just putting on my shoes. I wanted to get healthy and look better. Today my goals have changed. Now I want to give everything I have to glorify the Lord Jesus Christ; I want to turn heads, but not to me, but to him."

—Cameron Jackson

## TRACK THE UPS AND DOWNS

Planning is one thing, but recording how well you followed through with your intentions is quite another. To improve your fitness, you will want to slowly and progressively increase the intensity or duration of your exercise. For example, if you did ten push-ups last week to improve your fitness, you will want to try eleven push-ups the next time. If you walked a half mile on Monday, you will want to aim for a three-quarter-mile walk the next Monday.

Using *The Daniel Plan Journal* or App will help you to track your success as well as make note of any challenges or modifications you would like to make to your fitness program. Monitoring challenges allows you to identify any ongoing negative thoughts, behaviors, or patterns that may undermine your efforts to be more active. For example, let's say you promise yourself to exercise tomorrow morning, but tomorrow comes and goes, and you don't exercise. Instead of beating

## MIX IT UP

It takes your body only a few weeks to get used to a workout. Once something becomes routine for your muscles and metabolism, mental and physical plateaus become likely. The best way to keep your body from becoming bored is to mix it up! There are ten ways you can do that to help you maximize your fitness.

**1. Cross-train.** If you are a runner, you most likely love to run. If you are a swimmer, you most likely love to swim. Good for you! Remember, one of the essentials of lifelong fitness is to do what you love. But one thing to be aware of when you perform the same exercises over and over is that your body can become accustomed to the movement. So cross-training, a variety of movements or activities, enhances your overall performance and helps you in a number of ways:

- Prevents boredom
- Protects joints and body from overuse
- Extends longevity in sport or activity
- Prevents burnout[15]

It takes your body about two to four weeks to get used to a routine, so shake things up with cross-training and try something new every few weeks. Watch how your body responds.

**2. Increase the frequency.** If you have been successful at exercising for two days a week, give it a try to bump up your exercise to three days a week. By increasing the number of days you exercise, you will naturally challenge your body and create even greater fitness.

**3. Increase the intensity.** Increasing the speed, elevation, pace, or duration of your aerobic activity just a little bit could be just what you need to improve your cardiovascular fitness and boost your metabolism. For example, try interval training. If you are a walker, instead of walking at a steady pace, try walking at a moderate pace for one minute and then as fast as you can for one minute. You could even jog or run for the fast minute if you'd like. You may want to monitor your

yourself up, simply write down what thoughts, behaviors, or happened that day; then record two or three possible solution: next time.

We all know that when it comes to a regular exercise progi you don't plan it, it's probably not going to happen! It's true of important things in our lives, isn't it? So what's the best time to cise? The time you will do it — whether it's in the morning, du lunch, or after dinner. The key is to develop a routine that allows to make PLAY a regular part of your life.

The underlying question we encourage you to ask yourself you're putting together your fitness plan is, "What activities do I enjo and bring a smile to my face?" Think of ways you can integrate fun joy, laughter, devotion, excitement, and adventure into all aspects of your PLAY.

## Create a Toy Box

In your office or home, designate an area where you can keep fun fitness toys such as ...

| | |
|---|---|
| Basketball/soccer ball | Pedometer |
| Balance board | Resistance band |
| Hula hoop | Roller skates/blades |
| Foam roller | Stability ball |
| Jump rope | Wii Fit |

**Progress slowly.** Be conscious of progressing yourself slowly and alternating all aspects of your PLAY, and increase gradually. (That is, start with a ten-minute leisurely walk and then progress from there, or begin with three youthful strengthening movements, then move to four.) Small incremental progress is best, not only for your body, but also for your confidence.

heart rate as you challenge and change your intensity throughout your exercise.

Increase the number of reps, sets, or weight of the resistance of your youthful strength training movements. You can also perform movements that are total body, called "compound exercises," such as Kettlebell swings that use your upper and lower body. Another option is to manipulate the speed of your movements, either moving slowly — five seconds on the upward motion and five seconds on the downward motion — or exploding on the way up with each movement.

**4. Change your equipment or your environment.** If you are used to using dumbbells in your strength training, how about using a medicine ball or a stability ball to change things up? If you are used to going to the gym and waiting in line for a treadmill, an elliptical, or a bike, what about using one of those funny-looking machines that no one uses, such as the rowing machine, ski machine, or Versa climber? Why not grab that jump rope gathering dust in the corner of the gym?

Did you know you can burn almost two to three times more calories using total-body machines or exercises compared with slow walking on a treadmill? Plus, you will shake things up a bit by using different muscle groups in different ways. Also, if you are used to exercising indoors, go outside every few days. If you are an outside kind of person, why not give an aerobic or spinning class a try? Changing your scenery, meeting new people, and trying something different can be just what you need to keep your fitness routine fresh.

**5. Decrease your rest interval.** By decreasing the amount of time you rest in between exercises or sets, you will naturally increase the intensity of your workouts and cause your body to adapt and become stronger.

**6. Time your exercise routines.** For your next workout, try to beat your previous time. This type of training provides you with a tangible score to challenge yourself and cause your body to adapt to a new intensity.

**7. Give yourself a break.** Believe it or not, one of the worst things you can do to your body is to exercise too much with no rest. So one

### Buddy Up

What do Peyton Manning, Oprah Winfrey, Michael Jordan, George W. Bush, and Olympic Gold medalist Apolo Ohno all have in common? Your first thought might be success in their particular field. While that is true, all of them attribute their personal success to one thing: having a buddy, mentor, or coach who brought the best out of them. They each had someone in their lives who instructed, encouraged, pushed, trained, and taught them to pursue excellence, assisting them in reaching their dreams.

Similarly, when it comes to becoming Daniel Strong and attaining or maintaining your personal health and fitness goals, having a buddy who provides you with ongoing support, encouragement, and accountability is crucial to lasting personal progress. In twenty years of fitness training, Foy hasn't seen a more powerful step you can take toward better help than enlisting the support of a positive fitness buddy or buddies.

of the best things you can do for your body, especially if you are challenging yourself on a regular basis, is to take a break. Your body will thank you, and you will come back even more excited and ready to take your fitness to another level.

**8. Get a dog.** Scientists from the University of Western Australia found that people walk 48 minutes more per week after they get a dog.[16] Dogs are a natural fitness trainer — reminding you daily to take care of yourself, encouraging you to move, with every step and wag of their tail.

**9. Hire a personal trainer.** In providing professional program design, education, support, and motivation, monitoring progress, fine-tuning your program, and ensuring that proper technique is used during your training, a personal trainer could be just what you are looking for to get fit and stay fit.

**10. Exercise with others.** If you are used to exercising alone, try working out in a group setting to mix things up. Research has shown that when you work out with others, you will naturally increase the intensity of your workouts.[17] Try swapping your traditional exercise routine for a Pilates or spin class or boot camp or your traditional cardio for an active game or sport for one month to see how you feel.

We will talk more about the value and power of friends in chapter 7, but whether you are just beginning your fitness program or are looking for a boost to your current routine, having a fitness buddy can help you take your fitness to another level. So look for someone who has similar goals and interests to yours, has a similar schedule and fitness level, is dedicated and encouraging, and is someone you like spending time with. Supportive relationships, individuals who will be there for you, are the secret to becoming Daniel Strong.

### Reflect and Take a Step ...

The key to fitness is discovering movement that you enjoy. Don't worry about what other people are doing. Choose activities that bring you joy and put a smile on your face. Start with a small step in the right direction, and consider asking a friend to join you. You will be amazed how great you can feel.

# Chapter 6

# Focus

*Do not conform to the pattern of this world, but be transformed by the renewing of your mind (Romans 12:2).*

With one decision — an action made by your brain — you will begin a journey to wellness that will offer you increased energy, lower stress, and better sleep (among the many other benefits you have already read about). We want that one decision to last for a lifetime, which requires a renewed mind and sustained focus. In a world where so many distractions compete for your attention, it is more important than ever to stop the busyness in your head and focus on God's plan and priorities for your life. The bottom line is that whatever gets your attention gets you.

Unfortunately, it is the loss of focus that causes many people to cycle through hopeful starts and many failed stops as other things vie for their attention. We will help you optimize your brain health, renew your mind, increase your focus, and live with a purpose-driven mind-set.

All of the information in this book is designed to help you win the war between the thoughtful part of your brain that knows what you should do and your pleasure centers that always want gratification now. Your pleasure centers, deep in the brain, are always

> "To be made new in the attitude of your minds; and to put on the new self, created to be like God in true righteousness and holiness" (Ephesians 4:23 – 24).

looking for a good time: They crave the double cheeseburgers, will stand in line for the fresh cinnamon rolls, and convince you to stay

186 The **Daniel** Plan

on the couch in front of the TV for another hour instead of going for that run.

Left unchecked, your pleasure centers encourage thoughts such as

- We deserve it.
- Come on, let's have some fun!
- You're so uptight!
- Live a little.
- I already had one bowl of ice cream; just one more won't hurt.
- I'll be better tomorrow. I promise.

Without focus, your brain can ruin your health. To balance your pleasure centers, there is an area in the front part of your brain called the prefrontal cortex, which helps you think about what you do before you do it. It is the brain's brake that stops you from saying or doing stupid things. The prefrontal cortex is called the executive part of the brain because it acts like the boss at work and is involved with executive functions, such as focus, forethought, judgment, planning, and self-control. It thinks about your future, not just about what you want in the moment. Instead of thinking about the chocolate cake, it is the rational voice in your head that helps you avoid having a big belly, is concerned about your bulging medical bills, and has the ability to say no and mean it.

When your prefrontal cortex is strong, it reins in your pleasure centers so that you can enjoy life, but in a thoughtful, measured way. To get healthier and happier for the long run, it is critical to strengthen your brain.

# CHANGE YOUR BRAIN, CHANGE YOUR HEALTH

**YOUR BRAIN IS THE MOST AMAZING ORGAN.** Even though it is only 2 percent of your body's weight, it uses 20 to 30 percent of the calories you consume and 20 percent of the oxygen and blood flow in your body. It is the most expensive real estate in your body that requires the most resources. It has 100 billion nerve cells and more connections in it than there are stars in the universe.

When your brain works right, you work right. When your brain is troubled, you are much more likely to have trouble. With a healthy brain, people are happier and physically healthier, because they make better decisions. People with healthy brains are often wealthier and more successful because of those better decisions. (Are you beginning to see a pattern?) When the brain is not healthy, people are sadder, sicker, poorer, and less successful.

It is your brain that pushes you away from the table, telling you that you have had enough. It is your brain that gives you permission to have the third bowl of ice cream but chooses berries instead. If you want better health, strive to have a healthier brain. Ultimately, boosting brain health is about three specific strategies: (1) brain envy — you have to passionately care about your brain, (2) avoiding anything that hurts it, and (3) engaging in habits that boost its health.

*Brain envy* is a term Dr. Amen coined after looking at tens of thousands of brain SPECT scans of patients at the Amen Clinics. A brain SPECT (single photon emission computed tomography) scan evaluates blood flow and activity patterns in the brain. Dr. Amen's research clearly shows that healthy SPECT scans come from people who make smarter decisions and act in a way to bring health and goodness into their lives.

Yet few people ever think about their brains, much less care about them. We let little kids hit soccer balls with their heads, do dangerous

Saving My Brain

"A number of years ago my friend Doctor Cyrus Raji and his colleagues published a study reporting that as a person's weight went up, the size of his or her brain went down. That horrified me. I never want to purposefully do anything to harm the health of my brain. That information motivated me to get to a healthy weight so I could have a healthy mind.

"I first saw my brain in 1991 with the then-new technology of brain SPECT imaging. My brain looked older than I was. It motivated me to have what I call 'brain envy' and make radical changes with my health. I stopped drinking diet soda, started sleeping more than six hours a night, began exercising more, and focused on having more fun. I was vigilant about keeping sugar out of my diet, boosted my vegetable and lean protein intake, and made sure to always eat breakfast. Over time these things have become a natural part of my life."

—Dr. Amen

gymnastic routines, or play tackle football. In football and hockey, we cheer big hits, now known to cause lasting brain damage.

So why don't we care more about our brains? Because most people never see their brains. You can see the wrinkles in your face or the fat around your belly and do something when you don't like how they look, but the brain is different. If you could look at your brain, all of a sudden everything would change. You could see if yours is troubled and do something about it.

Since most people will not have the opportunity to look at their own brains, here are seven warning signs your brain may be in trouble. If you have any of these, it is time to develop brain envy and start taking much better care of it.

**1. Poor memory.** If your memory is worse than it was ten years ago, it is a sign your brain is struggling.

**2. Poor judgment/impulsiveness.** If you struggle with consistent problems of poor judgment or impulsive behavior, your brain may be troubled.

**3. Short attention span/distractibility.** Having a short attention span or being easily distracted could be a sign of brain dysfunction, meaning it is time to start taking better care of it.

**4. Depression.** From time to time all of us feel sad, but when sad or depressed feelings persist, it is called clinical depression and is usually associated with lower activity in the brain. Boosting brain function often has a very positive effect on mood. Many of The Daniel Plan choices have anti-depressant properties. Exercise, eating right, taking supplements such as fish oil, and learning not to believe every thought have been shown independently to boost mood.[1] If depression persists despite following The Daniel Plan strategies, please see a mental health care professional.

**5. Obesity or being overweight.** In studies at the Amen Clinics, we have found that as your weight goes up, your ability to think and reason goes down, which means that over time, if you don't get your weight under control, it will become harder for you to use your own good judgment.

**6. Low energy.** When people feel physically tired, it is often due to low brain function.

**7. Chronic insomnia/sleep apnea.** Another sign that your brain may be in trouble is a lack of sleep or sleep apnea. Research suggests that people who get less than seven hours of sleep at night have lower overall blood flow to the brain and poorer cognitive functioning.[2] Sleep apnea (snoring loudly, stopping breathing at night, or feeling chronically tired during the day) increases a person's risk for obesity, depression, and Alzheimer's disease. If you have insomnia or sleep apnea, it is critical to get them under control.

Start boosting your brain health by *avoiding anything that hurts the brain.* Illegal drugs, too much alcohol, brain trauma, environmental toxins, and infections are obvious. Now we also know that a poor diet, especially one high in sugar and simple carbohydrates, increases the risk of Alzheimer's disease fourfold.[3] Hypertension, diabetes, high blood sugar levels, chemotherapy, insomnia, and obesity can all damage the brain and lead to smaller brain volume and poorer cognitive abilities. Even high normal blood pressure and high normal fasting blood sugar levels lead to brain atrophy. In one large study, hypertensive individuals had 9 percent less brain volume than those who had normal blood pressure.[4]

There are now more than a hundred studies reporting that being overweight or obese damages brain tissue and function. Untreated depression, excessive stress, low hormone levels, such as thyroid or testosterone, and a lack of exercise or excessive exercise also hurt the brain.

When the two men first met, Pastor Warren told Dr. Amen that

### Finding Sleep

As Avery Parsons approached menopause, deteriorating sleep was at the top of her body's changes. With dramatic hormone shifts, Avery's sweet tooth was worse than ever. Getting through the afternoon required an extra latte or handfuls of chocolate or both! This not only spiked her blood sugar levels, but also created problems sleeping at night.

Recognizing the harmful cycle she had created, Avery turned to a list of Daniel Plan sleep tips to get back on track. Bit by bit, she improved her sleep. Cutting out the chocolate binges was the first priority. If she had any caffeine, she consumed it before noon. Avery also began preparing for sleep by turning off all electronics, dimming the lights, and putting on soft, relaxing music. Choosing to read a book helped relax her mind and send the message that it was nearing time for bed. Instead of relying on problematic sleep aids, she took 200–400mg of magnesium citrate to calm down her nervous system.

To start your own personal sleep hygiene routine, visit *danielplan.com* for a list of ideas.

he never felt motivated to get healthy for his heart and didn't really care about living longer or being "sexier." But when Pastor Warren heard that as his weight went up the size of his brain would go down, it motivated him to change. His motivation came from his brain — he wanted to protect his.

The last step to boosting brain health is to *engage in regular brain healthy habits*, including moderate physical exercise (which you read about in chapter 5), new learning, an amazing Daniel Plan – friendly eating plan (see chapter 10 for a 40-day meal plan), and simple supplements such as a multiple vitamin/mineral complex and omega 3 fatty acids. Omega 3 fatty acids improve mood and lessen anxiety, and the combination of vitamins B6, B12, and folic acid enhance memory and cognition.[5] Also, being at a healthy weight, being physically healthy, and getting adequate sleep enhances brain function, as does having regular prayer and stress management practices.

Think of the brain as a computer with both hardware and software. Once you optimize the physical functioning of the brain (its hardware), you optimize your mind (the software). But there is one more crucial behavior for your brain health — avoiding chronic stress.

## THE BRAIN AND STRESS

Stress is a normal part of everyday life. Bad traffic, a big deadline, a fight at home — hundreds of things can stress us out. When the event passes, so does the stress, and we can breathe a big sigh of relief. With chronic stress, however, there is no relief. Stemming from things like family discord, financial hardships, health issues, work conflicts, or school trouble, chronic stress is unrelenting. And it affects far too many of us. In a poll by the American Psychological Association, a whopping 80 percent of Americans say they feel significant stress.[6] That spells trouble for your brain and body.

Don't get us wrong — a *little* stress can be a good thing. When stress hits, the brain tells your body to start pumping out adrenaline (epinephrine) and cortisol, two hormones released by the adrenal glands. Within seconds your heart starts to pound faster, your breathing quickens, your blood courses faster through your veins, and your mind is on heightened alert. You're ready for anything — running away from a would-be mugger, giving a speech in front of a roomful of peers, or taking an exam.

These stress hormones are the primary chemicals of the fight-or-flight response. They are especially useful when you face an immediate threat, such as a rattlesnake in your front yard. The human brain is so advanced that merely imagining a stressful event will cause the body to react to the perceived threat as if it were actually happening. You can literally scare your body into a stress response. The brain is one powerful organ.

Brief surges of stress hormones are normal and beneficial. They motivate you to do a good job at work, study hard, or pay your bills on time. Those short bursts of adrenaline and cortisol are not the problem with stress. The problem is that for many of us, the stress reactions never stop. Traffic, bills, work, school, family conflict, not enough sleep, health issues, and jam-packed schedules keep us in a constant state of stress. Take note that it isn't just the bad stuff in life

## EVENTS THAT CAUSE STRESS

| NEGATIVE | POSITIVE |
| --- | --- |
| Death of a loved one | Starting a new job |
| Getting laid off | Marriage |
| Getting divorced | Having a baby |
| Unwanted pregnancy | Moving to a new home |
| Miscarriage | Getting a promotion |
| Being involved in a lawsuit | Transferring to a new school |
| Having health problems | Going to college |
| Having a sick relative | Having a bestselling book |
| Caring for an ailing family member | |
| Having a mental disorder or living with someone who has one | |

that causes stress. Even happy events, such as having a baby or getting a promotion, can be major stressors.

Chronic stress harms the brain. It constricts blood flow, which lowers overall brain function and prematurely ages your brain. A series of studies looked at long-term exposure to stress hormones, especially cortisol, and its effect on brain function in varying age groups. The older adults with continuously high levels of cortisol performed worse on memory tests than older adults with moderate-to-low cortisol levels. The older adults with high cortisol levels also had a 14 percent smaller hippocampus, the area involved with memory.[7] The hippocampus is part of the stress response system and sends out signals to halt the production of cortisol once a threat has vanished. But when the number of brain cells in the hippocampus is depleted, it no longer sends out this signal, which results in the release of even greater amounts of cortisol.

"Give all your worries and cares to God, for he cares about you" (1 Peter 5:7 NLT).

Excessive amounts of cortisol affect other areas of the brain too. Canadian researchers used functional brain imaging studies to show that exposure to stress hormones is associated with decreased activity, not only in the hippocampus, but also in the parts of the brain that control cognitive function and emotional balance.

When stress hurts your brain, it can also ravage your body. Your body responds to the way you think, feel, and act. Because of this brain-body connection, whenever you feel stressed, your body tries to tell you that something isn't right. For example, high blood pressure or a stomach ulcer might develop after a particularly stressful event, such as the death of a loved one. Chronic stress weakens your body's immune system, making you more likely to get colds, flu bugs, and other infections during emotionally difficult times. Stress has also been implicated in heart disease, hypertension, and even cancer.

Your boss is handing out pink slips. You just had a fight with your teenage daughter. You are late for an appointment. How do you react? You may try to calm your nerves with chocolate, ice cream, French fries, or potato chips (or all of the above). And there's a scientific reason why. Stress and cortisol are linked to increases in appetite and cravings for carbs and sweet stuff that can make you fat.

Living with stress on a daily basis makes you more likely to have issues with your weight for a number of other reasons. For example, chronic stress usually goes hand in hand with a lack of sleep. That pumps up cortisol production and throws appetite-control hormones

## Common Signs and Symptoms of Stress

- ☐ Frequent headaches or migraines
- ☐ Gritting or grinding teeth
- ☐ Stammering or tremors
- ☐ Neck ache, back pain, or muscle spasms
- ☐ Dry mouth or problems swallowing
- ☐ Frequent colds, infections, or herpes sores
- ☐ Stomach pain or nausea
- ☐ Difficulty breathing or sighing
- ☐ Chest pain or heart palpitations
- ☐ Poor sexual desire or performance
- ☐ Increased anger, frustration, or irritability
- ☐ Depression, frequent, or wild mood swings
- ☐ Increased or decreased appetite
- ☐ Insomnia, nightmares, or disturbing dreams
- ☐ Difficulty concentrating, racing thoughts
- ☐ Trouble learning new information
- ☐ Overreaction to petty annoyances
- ☐ Reduced work efficiency or productivity
- ☐ Excessive defensiveness or suspiciousness
- ☐ Constant fatigue or weakness
- ☐ Frequent use of over-the-counter drugs
- ☐ Excessive gambling or impulse buying[8]

out of balance. That should explain why you feel as if health flies out the window during stressful situations. So it's no surprise if you over-eat, crave sugary treats, and store more fat.

Since chronic stress can make you feel tired and achy, you are less inclined to exercise. Of course, you can't blame stress for all your poor health and weight gain, but you can see how easily it happens.

Chronic stress drains your emotional well-being and is associated with anxiety, depression, and Alzheimer's disease, all of which can affect your body. If you experience some form of emotional trauma — say you're involved in a car accident — your emotional system becomes very active, which can make you more upset and depressed. Then the battle of the bulge and unhappiness with your body can feel overwhelming.

Chronic stress can attack you at any stage of your life. When chronic stress hits you or someone in your circle, everyone suffers. You've heard of the trickle-down economic theory; there's also a trickle-down stress theory. When the boss is stressed out, everyone at work is stressed out. When your spouse is stressed out, everyone in the family is stressed out.

Stop the trickle-down effect and calm stress. Here are a few strategies that will boost your mood and your decision making.

**1. Pray on a regular basis.** Decades of research have shown that prayer calms stress and enhances brain function. Dr. Andrew Newberg at Thomas Jefferson University used brain SPECT imaging to study the neurobiology of prayer and meditation in those that dedicated time to those disciplines regularly. He found distinctive changes in brain activity as the mind went into a prayerful or meditative state. Specifically, activity decreased in the parts of the brain involved in generating a sense of three-dimensional orientation in space. They also found increased activity in the prefrontal cortex associated with attention span and thoughtfulness.[9] Prayer tunes people in, not out.

The benefits of prayer go far beyond stress relief. Studies have shown that it also improves attention and planning, reduces depression and anxiety, decreases sleepiness, and protects the brain from cognitive decline associated with normal aging.

As we mentioned in chapter 3, King David practiced biblical meditation and prayer. You can too, just about anywhere, anytime. If you're at work, you can simply close the door to your office, sit in your chair, close your eyes, and pray. At home, you can sit on the edge of your bed and spend a couple minutes calming your mind and focusing on God. The Bible says, "Whatever is true, whatever is noble, whatever is right, whatever is pure, whatever is lovely, whatever is admirable — if anything is excellent or praiseworthy — think about such things" (Philippians 4:8).

God wants us to think deeply on his goodness and loveliness. This is biblical meditation. The Bible says, "In repentance and rest is your salvation, in quietness and trust is your strength" (Isaiah 30:15). You need to regularly, repeatedly set time aside to quiet yourself and refocus your thoughts on the greatness and power of God.

Besides growing your relationship with God and building a foundation for spiritual health, prayer offers many health and stress-relief benefits. Physicians Larry Dossey (*Healing Words*), Dale Matthews (*The Faith Factor*), and others have written books outlining the scientific evidence of the medical benefits of prayer and other meditation.[10] Some of these benefits include reduced feelings of stress, lower cholesterol levels, improved sleep, reduced anxiety and depression, fewer headaches, relaxed muscles, and longer life spans. People who pray or read the Bible every day are 40 percent less likely to suffer from hypertension than others.[11]

A 1998 Duke University study of 577 men and women hospitalized for physical illness showed that the more patients used positive spiritual coping strategies (seeking spiritual support from friends and religious leaders, having faith in God, praying), the lower their level of depressive symptoms and the higher their quality of life.[12] A 1996 survey of 269 family physicians found that 99 percent believed prayer, meditation, or other spiritual and religious practices can be helpful in medical treatment; more than half said they currently incorporate these practices into treatment of patients.[13]

> "You will keep in perfect peace all who trust in you, all whose thoughts are fixed on you!" (Isaiah 26:3 NLT).

**2. Learn to delegate.** It seems as if being busy is a sort of badge of honor. Ask anyone what they have planned for the day, and it's likely they will respond by telling you how incredibly busy they are. "I'm finishing a project for work, hosting a dinner party, making the kids' costumes for the school play, volunteering at church, and going to my book group." Phew! It can stress you out just thinking about all that.

### Ten Names of God to Dwell On

1. *Jehovah Rapha* — the God who heals, who makes healthful
2. *El Roiy* — the God who sees me
3. *Jehovah Jirah* — the Lord who provides
4. *El Shadai* — All sufficient one, Lord God Almighty
5. *Jehovah Nissi* — the Lord our banner of loving protection
6. *Jehovah Oz* — the Lord my strength
7. *Adonai* — the Sovereign Lord God
8. *Jehovah Shammah* — the Lord is there
9. *Jehovah Shalom* — Our perfect peace
10. *Jehovah Raah* — the Lord my shepherd

News flash! You don't have to accept every invitation, take on every project, or volunteer for every activity that comes your way. Two of the greatest life skills you can learn are the art of delegation and the ability to say no. When someone asks you to do something, a good first response would be, "Let me think about it." Then you can take the time to process the request to see if it fits with your schedule, desires, and goals. When you have too much on your plate, delegate.

**3. Listen to soothing music.** Music has healing power that can bring peace to a stressful mind. Of course, it depends on the type of music you listen to. Listening to uplifting music that reminds you of God's truth can have a calming effect and reduce stress and calm anxiety.

**4. Consider calming scents.** The scent of lavender has been used since ancient times for its calming, stress-relieving properties. This popular aroma has been the subject of countless research studies, which show that it reduces cortisol levels and promotes relaxation and stress reduction. Add a few drops of lavender oil to your bath or set dried lavender in your bedroom. Many other scents, such as geranium, rose, cardamom, sandalwood, and chamomile, are considered to have a calming effect that reduces stress.

**5. Take a calming supplement.** Some supplements may be helpful in soothing stress, but take these under the supervision of a health care professional.

*B vitamins* help the brain affect mood and thinking.

*L-Theanine* is an amino acid mainly found naturally in the green tea plant. It penetrates the brain and produces significant increases in the anti-depressant neurotransmitters serotonin and/or dopamine concentrations. *Note:* Pregnant women and nursing mothers should avoid L-theanine supplements.

*GABA:* Gama-aminobutyric acid (GABA) works in much the same way as anti-anxiety drugs and anticonvulsants. This means it has a calming effect for people who struggle with temper, irritability, and anxiety, whether these symptoms relate to anxiety.

**6. Laugh more.** There is a growing body of scientific literature suggesting that laughter counteracts stress and is good for the immune system. It's no joke! One study of cancer patients found that laughter reduced stress and improved cell activity associated with increased resistance to the disease.[14] According to University of California – Irvine's Professor Lee Berk, "If we took what we know about the medical benefits of laughter and bottled it up, it would require FDA approval." Laughter lowers the flow of dangerous stress hormones. Laughter also eases digestion and soothes stomachaches, a common symptom of chronic stress. Plus, a good rollicking guffaw increases the release of endorphins, which make you feel better and more relaxed. Laughter truly may be the best medicine when it comes to stress relief.

> "A cheerful heart is good medicine" (Proverbs 17:22).

The average child laughs hundreds of times a day. The average adult laughs only a dozen times a day. Inject more humor into your everyday life. Watch comedies (which could be a helpful form of TV), go to humorous plays, read joke books, and swap funny stories with your friends and family.

We can't stress enough (pun intended) how important it is to learn to laugh at yourself too. When you drop the milk jug and it goes splashing across the kitchen floor, when you call a business associate by the wrong name, or when you stumble over your words while teaching a class, be the first to chuckle. When you stop taking yourself so seriously, your stress levels will subside.

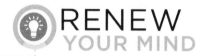

# RENEW
## YOUR MIND

**NOW THAT YOU KNOW** how to optimize your brain health, we want to focus on the power center of your brain — your thoughts.

Philippians 4:8 (see page 196) is one of the most powerful, emotionally healing verses in the Bible. One of the cornerstones to success on The Daniel Plan is to reign over your moment-by-moment thoughts, so that with God's help you can stay in control of your behavior.

Neuroscience teaches us that every time you have a thought, your brain releases chemicals that make you feel good or bad. Thoughts exert a powerful influence over your life and body. Whenever you have a happy, hopeful, or optimistic thought, your brain releases chemicals that raise your spirits and encourage you to feel good. Positive thoughts exert a physical response and have the power to immediately relax and soothe your body. They tend to warm your hands, relax your muscles, calm and soothe your breathing, and help your heart beat in a healthier rhythm.

Try this exercise now: Take a minute, close your eyes, and think of the last time you felt truly loved. When most people do this exercise, they feel a deep sense of happiness and physical relaxation.

The opposite is also true. When you have an angry, anxious, hopeless, or helpless thought, your brain releases chemicals that stress your body and disrupt how you feel both physically and emotionally. Take a minute, close your eyes, and think of the last time you felt really angry. How did that make you feel? Most people feel tense, their breathing becomes shallower, their hands become colder, and they feel angry and unhappy. Now go back to the first exercise before you continue reading!

Thoughts are automatic. They just happen. They are based on complex chemical reactions and information from the past. And what most people don't know is that thoughts are sneaky and they lie. They

## Think on God's Character

**God is all-powerful:** "Ah, Sovereign LORD, you have made the heavens and the earth by your great power and outstretched arm. Nothing is too hard for you" (Jeremiah 32:17).

**God is love:** "For I am convinced that neither death nor life, neither angels nor demons, neither the present nor the future, nor any powers, neither height nor depth, nor anything else in all creation, will be able to separate us from the love of God that is in Christ Jesus our Lord" (Romans 8:38–39).

**God is all-knowing:** "Before a word is on my tongue, you, LORD, know it completely. You hem me in behind and before, and you lay your hand upon me. Such knowledge is too wonderful for me, too lofty for me to attain" (Psalm 139:4–6).

**God is merciful:** "Therefore, there is now no condemnation for those who are in Christ Jesus, because through Christ Jesus the law of the Spirit who gives life has set you free from the law of sin and death" (Romans 8:1–2).

**God is faithful:** "Because of the LORD's great love we are not consumed, for his compassions never fail. They are new every morning; great is your faithfulness" (Lamentations 3:22–23).

lie a lot. It is often these uninvestigated thoughts that provide the emotional fuel for anger, anxiety, depression, and unhealthy behaviors such as overeating.

Plus, if you never question your erroneous, negative thoughts, you believe them 100 percent and then you act as if the lies in your head are true. For example, if you think your husband never listens to you, even though he has on many occasions, you act as if he doesn't, and you feel justified in yelling at him. If you think you are a failure, even though you have had many successes, you are more likely to give up easily.

Over the last forty years, mental health practitioners have developed cognitive behavioral therapy to help people rein in and control their erroneous thought patterns. When you correct negative thought patterns, it is an effective treatment for anxiety disorders, depression, relationship problems, and even overeating. Researchers from Sweden found that people who were trained to talk back to their negative thoughts lost seventeen pounds in ten weeks and continued to lose weight over eighteen months, proving this technique works long term.[15]

To get and stay healthy, start by noticing your thoughts and questioning them. Whenever you feel sad, mad, nervous, or out of control, ask yourself if they are really true. It is often the little lies we tell ourselves that keep us fat, depressed, and feebleminded. Being overweight or unhappy is as much a "thinking disorder" as it is an eating or mood disorder.

### IS IT TRUE?

"Is it true?" Carry these three words with you everywhere you go. They can interrupt your thoughts and short circuit an episode of bingeing, depression, or even panic. One of our participants weighed 425 pounds when he first joined The Daniel Plan. When one of the doctors asked him about his weight, he said that he had no control over his appetite. That was his automatic response, "I have no control."

"Is it true?" the doctor asked. "You really have NO control over your eating?"

The man paused, then said, "No. That really isn't true, I do have some control."

"But just by thinking that you have no control, you have just given yourself permission to eat anything you want at any time you want," the doctor replied. It is the little lies that you tell yourself — such as "I have no control" or "It is my genetics" — that steal your health.

One of the most important steps in getting healthy in a lasting way is to get control of your mind. Whenever you feel anxious, sad, obsessive, or out of control, write down the thoughts that are going through your head. Recording thoughts helps to get them out of your head. Then ask yourself if the thoughts make sense or are really true. For example, if you hear yourself thinking, *I have no control*, write that

## Common Lies

Here are some of the common little lies we have heard The Daniel Plan participants say:

"I can't eat healthy because I travel." We are amused by this one, because all of us — Pastor Warren, Dr. Hyman, Dr. Amen, and Sean Foy — travel a lot. It just takes a little forethought.

"My whole family is fat; it is in my genes." Genes account for only 20 to 30 percent of your health. The vast majority of health problems are driven by bad decisions. Many healthy people have the genes that increase the risk of obesity, but they do not make the decisions that make it likely to happen.

"I can't afford to get healthy." Being sick is always more expensive than getting healthy.

"I can't find the time to work out." The extra energy exercise will help you be even more efficient in the long run and save you time.

"It's Easter ... Memorial Day ... July 4th, Labor Day, Thanksgiving, Christmas, Friday, Saturday, Sunday, Monday, Tuesday, Wednesday, or Thursday." There is always an excuse to hurt yourself.

down. Then ask yourself, "Is it true? Is that thought really true?" If not, replace that negative, false thought with correct information.

When you stop believing these lies and replace them with accurate thinking and God's truth and promises, your response to life events will shift, and you will feel less stressed and more hopeful. Instead of worrying about tomorrow, you can linger on truths such as Jeremiah 29:11: " 'For I know the plans I have for you,' declares the LORD, 'plans to prosper you and not to harm you, plans to give you hope and a future.' "

## HOW WE DISTORT OUR THOUGHTS

Over the years, therapists have identified a number of negative thoughts that keep people stuck in bad habits:

**1. Overgeneralization.** This usually involves thoughts with words such as *always, never, every time,* or *everyone* and makes a situation out to be worse than it really is. Here are some examples:

*I have always been fat; it will never change.*

### Truth to Combat Lies

"So do not fear, for I am with you; do not be dismayed, for I am your God. I will strengthen you and help you; I will uphold you with my righteous right hand" (Isaiah 41:10).

"But [God] said to me, 'My grace is sufficient for you, for my power is made perfect in weakness.' Therefore I will boast all the more gladly about my weaknesses, so that Christ's power may rest on me" (2 Corinthians 12:9).

"Come to me, all you who are weary and burdened, and I will give you rest. Take my yoke upon you and learn from me, for I am gentle and humble in heart, and you will find rest for your souls. For my yoke is easy and my burden is light" (Matthew 11:28–30).

"The LORD your God is with you, the Mighty Warrior who saves. He will take great delight in you; in his love he will no longer rebuke you, but will rejoice over you with singing" (Zephaniah 3:17).

"Let us then approach God's throne of grace with confidence, so that we may receive mercy and find grace to help us in our time of need" (Hebrews 4:16).

"Take delight in the LORD, and he will give you the desires of your heart" (Psalm 37:4).

*Every time I get stressed, I have to eat something.*

*I don't like any of the foods that are good for me.*

Overgeneralizations creep into your mind and have an immediate, negative effect on your mood. Overgeneralizations make you believe you have no control over your actions and behaviors and that you are incapable of changing them.

**2. Thinking with your feelings.** These negative thoughts occur when you have a feeling about something and you assume your feeling is correct. Feelings are complex and are often rooted in powerful memories from the past. Feelings, like thoughts, can lie too. These thoughts usually begin with the words "I feel." For example:

*I feel like a failure.*

*I feel God has abandoned me.*

*I feel hungry and must eat or I will get sick.*

Whenever you have a strong negative feeling, check it out. Look for the evidence behind the feeling. Is it based on events or experiences from the past?

**3. Predicting the future.** Predicting the worst in a situation causes an immediate sense of anxiety, which can trigger cravings for sugar or refined carbs and make you feel that you need to eat to calm your nerves. What makes future-telling thoughts so toxic is that your mind tends to make happen what it sees.

*Healthy food will be expensive, taste like cardboard, and won't fill me up.*

*I can't change my habits for the long term.*

*My spouse or my kids will never do this with me.*

**4. Blame.** When you blame something or someone else for the problems in your life, you become a victim of circumstances, as though you can't do anything to change your situation. Blaming thoughts can keep you unhealthy and unhappy. Be honest and ask yourself if you have a tendency to say things such as ...

"It's your fault I'm out of shape because you won't exercise with me."

"It's not my fault I eat too much; my mom taught me to clean my plate."

"If restaurants didn't give such big servings, I wouldn't be so overweight."

One of the participants of The Daniel Plan said he was fat because everyone in his family was overweight. It was just his genetics. "Is that true?" we asked. "This really doesn't have anything to do with how much you eat?" He paused and said, "No, it's really not true. In fact, not all my siblings are overweight."

Whenever you begin a sentence with "It's your fault that I ...," it can ruin your life. These thoughts make you a victim. And when you're a victim, you become powerless to change your behavior.

**5. Denial.** These thoughts prevent you from seeing the truth.

*I have plenty of time to work on getting healthy.*

*If I don't buy sugar cereals, my kids won't eat breakfast in the morning.*

*I can stop consuming alcohol anytime I want. I just don't want to quit.*

*I only overeat when I'm stressed, not every day.*

Now it's time to learn how to develop a little mental discipline and turn your negative thinking patterns into positive, accurate, healthy thinking, similar to how we encouraged you with spiritual discipline in chapter 3. We want you to learn how to discipline your thoughts to be honest and helpful. A 2010 study found that a twelve-week program designed to change thinking patterns helps binge eaters stop their negative eating behaviors.[16]

**6. Focusing on the negative.** Many people are masterful in finding something negative to say about any situation. This negative cognition takes a positive experience and taints it.

*I wanted to lose thirty pounds in ten weeks, but I have only lost
  eight pounds. I'm a complete failure.*

*I went to the gym and did a hard workout, but the guy on the bike
  next to me was talking the whole time, so I'm never going back
  there.*

*I started eating two servings of vegetables a day, but I should be
  eating five for optimal health, so why bother?*

Putting a positive spin on your thoughts leads to positive changes
in your brain that will help you stick with healthier choices. For example, here's how you could think about these same situations:

*I have already lost eight pounds and have changed my lifestyle,
  so I will continue to lose weight until I reach my goal of losing
  thirty pounds.*

*After working out, I had a lot more energy for the rest of the day.*

*Eating two servings of vegetables a day is better than none.*

### Banning the Negativity

When Solange Montoya started The Daniel Plan with two
friends, she was hoping to change more than her weight
and how her clothes fit. She knew there was more to lifelong
health. And there was!

"So many insecurities and all this negative self-talk come
when you don't feel like you can do this physically," she says.
"But there was such a change when I had that energy and
[started thinking positively instead of negatively]. I just feel
like, *Wow, God, there's nothing now that I don't want to do for
you.* The excuses just kind of started to melt away, more so
than the weight. There's this freedom that comes with me now
wanting to get out there and live my life—not just for me, but
for my kids, for God, and for other people."

Whenever you feel sad, mad, nervous, or out of control, identify which of the six types of the negative thoughts you are engaging in. Challenge the negative thoughts by finding and stating the truth. This takes away their power and gives you control over your thoughts, moods, and behaviors.

## ELIMINATE NEGATIVE THOUGHT PATTERNS

| NEGATIVE THOUGHT | TYPE | ELIMINATE IT WITH TRUTH |
|---|---|---|
| Every time I get stressed, I eat something. | Overgeneralization | Actually, many times when I am stressed I don't overeat. I will develop ten alternative things to do when stressed so I don't overeat. |
| I'll never lose weight. | Predicting the future | I've never tried to lose weight. If I change my behavior and adopt The Daniel Plan, I can be successful like many, many others. |
| | | |
| | | |
| | | |
| | | |

## GRATITUDE

Another way to discipline your mind — that feels good — is to bring your attention to the things you are grateful for in your life. Research reveals that being consistently grateful will have a positive effect on your health.[17] God designed us in such a way that gratitude promotes healing.

A Yale University research study evaluated more than 2,000 veterans between the ages of 60 and 96 to assess which traits helped them age successfully.[18] Gratitude and purpose were the most significant traits associated with successful aging. Your attitude matters.

Another study, from the University of California – Davis, examined the effect of a grateful outlook on psychological and physical well-being. Participants were randomly assigned to one of three experimental conditions. They kept weekly or daily journals to write about hassles, gratitude, or neutral events. They also recorded their moods, coping behaviors, health behaviors, physical symptoms, and overall life appraisals. The grateful group exhibited the most heightened well-being.[19]

> "Rejoice always, pray continually, give thanks in all circumstances; for this is God's will for you in Christ Jesus" (1 Thessalonians 5:16–18).

Where you bring your attention determines how you feel, and feeling grateful is a joyful place to be. This mind-set also helps your faith as you focus on God's gifts to you. It helps you eat right as you focus on being grateful for the ability to eat delicious, healthy food that serves your body. It helps you maintain your fitness level as you feel grateful for the ability to move your body. And it helps your friends as you notice what you like about them more than what you don't like.

Gratefulness actually helps your brain work better. Psychologist Noelle Nelson in her book *The Power of Appreciation in Everyday Life*

### Morning Ritual

The first thing on Dr. Amen's master to-do list, the first thing he sees each day, is his gratitude list. Rather than just writing down a few things, he keeps a running tab on what he is grateful for, looks at it every day, and adds to it as joyful moments occur.

described a study where she had a brain SPECT scan twice. The first time she was scanned after thirty minutes of meditating on all the things she was thankful for in her life. Then she was scanned several days later after focusing on the major fears in her life. After the appreciation exercise, her brain looked very healthy. The scan taken after she focused on her fears looked very different. Activity in two parts of her brain had significantly dropped. Her cerebellum completely shut down.[20]

The other area of Dr. Nelson's brain that was affected was the temporal lobes, especially the one on the left. The temporal lobes are involved with mood, memory, and temper control. Problems in this part of the brain are associated with some forms of depression, but also dark thoughts, violence, and memory problems. Practicing gratitude literally helps you have a brain to be grateful for.

Here is a helpful exercise: Write down three things you are grateful for every day. The act of writing down your grateful thoughts helps to bring your attention to them to enhance your brain. Research from University of Pennsylvania psychologist Martin Seligman demonstrates that when people do this exercise, they notice a significant positive difference in their level of happiness in just three weeks.[21] Other researchers have also found that people who express gratitude on a regular basis are healthier, more optimistic, make more progress toward their goals, have a greater sense of well-being, and are more helpful to others. Doctors who regularly practice gratitude are actually better at making the correct diagnoses on their patients.

Notice the connection Philippians 4:6 – 7 makes between gratitude and peace of mind: "Do not be anxious about anything, but in every situation, by prayer and petition, *with thanksgiving*, present your requests to God. And the *peace of God*, which transcends all understanding, will guard your hearts and your minds in Christ Jesus." It's not enough just to present your requests to God. Do it with thanksgiving if you also want peace of mind.

## THE B STUFF

At the turn of the century, a shoe company sent a representative to Africa. He wired back, "I'm coming home. No one wears shoes here." Another company sent their representative, and he sold thousands of shoes. He wired back to his company, "Business is fantastic. No one has ever heard of shoes here." Both reps perceived the same situation from markedly different perspectives, and they obtained dramatically different results.

We are not controlled by events or people, but by the perceptions we make of them. All of us have experienced a fair amount of criticism for our work over the years, as we have tried to do things differently in our fields of expertise. We had the option of feeling hurt, demoralized, and stopping the work we believed in. Or we had the option of realizing that anyone who does something in a different way is likely to be criticized. It was just part of the territory of trying to make a difference.

Perception is the way we interpret ourselves and the world around us. Our five senses take in the world, but perception occurs as our brains process the incoming information through our feeling filters.

> "Life is 10 percent what happens to me and 90 percent how I react to it."
> — Charles Swindoll

Our perception of the outside world is based on our inside world. For example, when we are feeling tired, we are much more likely to overeat or snap at our spouse or children than when we are rested.

The view that we take of a situation has more reality than the situation itself. Noted psychiatrist Richard Gardner, M.D., has said that the world is like a Rorschach test, where a person is asked to describe what he or she sees in 10 ink blots that mean absolutely nothing. What you see in the ink blot is based on your inner view of the world. Therefore, it is how you perceive situations, rather than the actual situations themselves, that cause you to react.

*If A is the actual event and B is how we interpret or perceive the event, then C is how we react to the event: A + B = C.*

Other people or events (A) trigger our initial feelings, but it is our interpretation or perception (B) of those people or events that causes how we eventually feel or act (C). For example, suppose you worked hard to bring a healthy meal to the church function, but someone made a negative comment, such as, "It looks so healthy, it probably tastes like cardboard." That is A, or what actually happened. You might think, *She hates me! My efforts were a waste of time and money,* or *Every time I try to do something good, it fails.* Your interpretation of her comment is B. Then you feel terrible and withdraw from further efforts to get healthy and be involved. Your reaction is C.

If, on the other hand, your thoughts about her comments (A) go in a different direction, and you think, *Poor woman, she is judging the food without even tasting it* (B), you might then encourage her to taste it (C) or allow others to rave about it (C). Your thoughts about the comments determine how you feel, not the comments themselves.

> Our perceptions are one of the largest influences on what dictates our behavior.

On this path toward a healthier life, we encourage you to identify your perceptions, starting with yourself. Do you see yourself as the child of God you are, dearly loved by the one who gave his life for you (John 3:16)? We too seldom treat ourselves with the love of God or even the love of a good parent. When we make a mistake, we might behave in an abusive manner toward ourselves. We may overeat, belittle ourselves, and feel hopeless. When children make mistakes, good parents don't belittle or abuse them; rather, they help them learn from their mistakes.

Just questioning your thoughts and perceptions and then filtering them through a loving God and honest mind will make a huge difference in your life, happiness, and health.

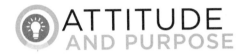

# ATTITUDE
## AND PURPOSE

**ANOTHER CRITICAL "FOCUS" STRATEGY** is your attitude toward failure. We have something very important to tell you that is absolutely essential for your mind. On The Daniel Plan you cannot fail — because you start it as a forty-day journey and then get to see changes gradually unfold over your lifetime. In The Daniel Plan — or in life, for that matter — no one just gets better. You get better … have a slip up … move forward…. Setbacks *and* comebacks are part of the journey, and graciousness must be part of both.

When you make a mistake, just make a U-turn. Do you have a GPS device on your phone or in your car? When you make a wrong turn, the GPS doesn't call you an idiot. It just tells you where to make the next legal U-turn. If you pay attention to your mistakes, such as that you went too long between meals, didn't sleep, or failed to plan, they can be your best teachers. Very soon you find yourself in a new place where you have dramatically improved both your brain and your body.

## CHANGE OCCURS IN STEPS

The diagram on the top of the next page is often used for participants in research studies.

We usually think of failure as a negative experience. But wise people know how to take advantage of failure. They learn from it. They make the most of it. They use it as an education.

Supposedly, Thomas Edison had about 1,000 failures when he was inventing the lightbulb. When asked by a reporter how it felt to fail so many times, Edison is said to have replied, "I didn't fail one thousand times. The lightbulb was an invention with one thousand steps."

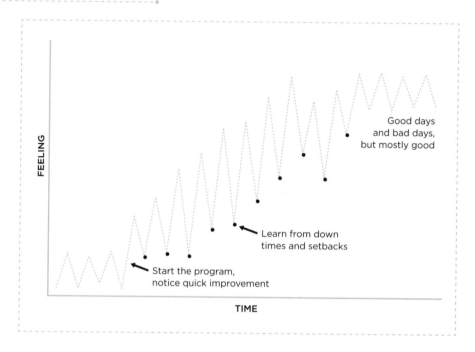

God uses failure to educate us. Mistakes are simply learning experiences, and there are some things we learn only through failure. So some of us are highly educated!

How do you learn to become a success? By learning what doesn't work and not doing it anymore. Saddleback Church has done more things that didn't work than did. Every staff member and minister at the church makes at least one good mistake a week. If we're not making any mistakes, we're not growing. But we aren't afraid of failure. The freedom from the fear of failure is the freedom to grow.

### Good Data

Setbacks help you identify your most vulnerable moments. We do not want you to be victims of your failures, but rather to study them just as a scientist would do. Be curious. We like saying, "Turn bad days into good data."

Your setbacks can even reaffirm your faith. It may surprise you to know that admitting your hopelessness to God can be a statement of faith. King David said, "I believed in you, so I said, 'I am deeply troubled, LORD.' In my anxiety I cried out to you" (Psalm 116:10 – 11 NLT).

David's frankness actually reveals a deep faith: First, he believed in God. Second, he believed God would listen to his prayer. Third, he believed God would let him say how he felt and still love him.

Regardless of your circumstances and how you feel, focus on who God is — his unchanging nature. Remind yourself what you know to be eternally true about God: He is good, he loves me, he is for me. He knows my struggles and my circumstances, and I know he has a good plan for my life.

## Simple Rules for Vulnerable Times

One tip we have found helpful for people who study their failures is to create simple rules for vulnerable times, such as ...

- Eat healthy foods before bad ones.
- Eat veggies first.
- Eat before you go to the ballgame to avoid being tempted by the caramel apples.
- When tempted, take a walk, repeat a poem, drink a glass of water.

Be aware of the impulse and then focus on something else until the impulse goes away.

Failure can also be motivational. A lot of times we change, not when we see the light, but when we feel the heat. When you fail, maybe God is trying to get your attention and saying, "I want you to go in a new direction."

Failure does not automatically grow your character. Failure only builds your character when you respond to it correctly, when you learn from it, when you grow from it, when you say, "What didn't work here, and what can I change?" When you think about failure and setbacks like this, your heart softens. Failure makes you less judgmental and helps you be a little more sympathetic to people around you.

## BE PURPOSE DRIVEN

The entrance to the Saddleback Campus in Lake Forest, California, starts on "Purpose Drive" for a reason. In our first Daniel Plan rally, we had our participants fill out an exercise plan to help them clearly define their vision or mission, a written purpose statement to help them focus all of their thoughts, words, and actions. Why? Your amazing brain makes what it sees happen. Seeing success in your mind makes it more likely to happen — as does seeing failure.

So we would like you to do this exercise too. Write out your major goals and purpose. Use the following headings:

- Faith
- Food
- Fitness
- Focus
- Friends

The five Essentials are separated in order to encourage you to have a more balanced approach to life. Burnout occurs when your life becomes unbalanced and you overextend yourself in one area while ignoring the others.

Next to each heading write what you believe God wants for you and what you want for yourself. Be positive and use the first person. Write your purpose with confidence and the expectation that with God's power it can happen. If you need to, work on it over several days. After you finish with the initial draft (you will frequently want to update it), place this list where you can see it every day, such as on your refrigerator, in your phone, by your bedside, or as your desktop wallpaper.

## Chuck's Purpose-Driven Exercise

Chuck is a manager at a local bank. He is married with three children. He had been recently diagnosed with diabetes and hypertension when he came to The Daniel Plan rally. Here is what he wrote down for his purpose-driven exercise:

"**Faith**—To live close to God, to seek his purpose for my life, trust God in the moment, pray daily, and attend church regularly.

"**Food**—Focus on food that serves my body and spirit. With the recent diagnoses of diabetes and hypertension, this is more critical now than ever before. I consume only whole, high-quality food, plenty of water, lean protein, healthy fats, low-glycemic, high-fiber carbohydrates, and an abundance of colorful fruits and vegetables. I eat often enough to maintain a stable blood sugar to avoid cravings.

"**Fitness**—My body is the temple of the Holy Spirit. I treat it with love and respect, which means exercising it on a regular basis, at least four times a week.

"**Friends**—Stay connected to those I love and be a role model of health and wholeness. I want to have a kind, caring, loving relationship with my wife and be a firm, kind, positive, predictable presence in my children's lives, and to take time to maintain and nurture my friendships.

"**Focus**—Focus on brain envy and brain healthy habits, SMART goals, my motivation, accurate, honest thoughts, gratitude, the right attitude toward failure, and journaling."

Whenever you do a behavior over and over, such as reading your purpose-driven exercise daily, it actually develops and strengthens specific pathways in the brain. The purpose-driven exercise can become the guidepost for all of your thoughts, feelings, and actions.

## SMART GOALS

We also want you to make SMART (Specific, Measurable, Attainable, Relevant, and Time-Bound) goals — similar to what we talked about in chapter 5 on fitness — for the other areas of your life that you wish to improve. Proverbs 4:26 says, "Give careful thought to the paths for your feet and be steadfast in all your ways."

Pastor Warren teaches that goal setting, like prayer and spending time alone with God, is a spiritual discipline. In fact, goals can be an act of stewardship or worship where you say, "God, I want to make the most of what I've been given" or "God, I give you back the life you've given to me, and I want to go in your direction."

Some people think, *I'm not going to plan; I'm just going to trust God and go with the flow.* Yes, we should trust God. But we should also plan, because the Bible says God plans. "God plans to bring all of history to its goal in Christ" (Ephesians 1:10 paraphrased). Notice that God doesn't just sit around and let things happen. And we have the choice to follow his lead.

**Specific** goals are those that are clear and unambiguous. This is where you tell your brain exactly what is expected and why it is important. A specific goal usually answers five "W" questions:

- *What:* What do I want to accomplish? For example, to lose 30 pounds.
- *Why:* Specific reasons, purposes, or benefits of accomplishing the goal. For example, to get truly healthy, have better energy, and be physically able to do God's purpose in my life.
- *Who:* Who is involved? For example, me, but it will also involve those closest to me.
- *Where:* Identify a location. For example, at home and everywhere I go.
- *Which:* Identify the requirements and constraints. For example, faith, food, fitness, focus, and friends.

To set specific goals, you need to know the difference between pressures and priorities. You need to know the difference between activity and achievement, between what's urgent and what's important. You need to know what matters most. If you focus your energy on goals that aren't God-directed, your energy won't have much power. Energy that is focused has enormous power. Paul modeled this in 1 Corinthians 9:26: "Therefore I do not run like someone running aimlessly; I do not fight like a boxer beating the air."

**Measurable** emphasizes the need for tangible benchmarks. If a goal is not measurable, it is not possible to know whether you are making progress toward it. Measuring your progress helps you stay on track and keeps you excited. A measurable goal will usually answer questions such as "how much? By when?"

**Attainable** means the goals need to be realistic, even though dreams can be big. Extreme goals usually invite failure and frustration. When you identify goals that are most important to you, your brain begins to figure out ways to make them come true.

At the same time, you must also realize that attainable doesn't mean only the goals you can accomplish in your own power. Goals can stretch your faith and affirm your trust in God. If you can do it in your own power, then you don't really need any faith. Saddleback Church is the story of ordinary people setting and attempting big goals in faith and then watching God do it.

**Relevant** means you choose goals that matter. The goal of "surf 100 websites by 9:00 p.m." may be specific, measurable, attainable, and time-bound, but lacks relevance. A relevant goal answers yes to these questions: Does this seem worthwhile? Is this the right time? Does this match your other efforts/ needs?

> Goals keep you moving forward when you feel like giving up. They are like magnets that pull you forward and give you hope.

Being relevant also means your goals are relevant to God and bring him glory. Any goal that brings you closer to him and makes you want to serve him and others is a goal that matters. The apostle Paul encouraged us to "make it our goal to please him, whether we are at home in the body or away from it" (2 Corinthians 5:9).

**Time-bound** stresses the importance of attaining the goal within a certain time frame. A commitment to a deadline helps you focus your efforts on completion of the goal on or before the due date. Time-bound criteria help you focus your efforts.

Here are some examples of SMART goals:

1. Walk as if I am late 4 times a week for 45 minutes with my walking partner.
2. Do a complete kitchen cleanse (removing all unhealthy food) this week.
3. Spend one night a week with friends reading and discussing The Daniel Plan material. Call in between meetings for encouragement and accountability.
4. Spend 5 to 10 minutes a day journaling my progress.
5. From this moment forward, focus on eating The Daniel Plan – approved foods 90 percent of the time.

Work toward SMART goals that give your brain and mind clear direction and focus on what is important.

## KNOW YOUR MOTIVATION

In order to get and stay healthy, it is critical for you to know *why* it is important. What drives your desire to be healthy?

Is it because it is God's will for you to take care of your body? Consider 1 Corinthians 6:19 – 20: "Do you not know that your bodies are temples of the Holy Spirit, who is in you, whom you have received from God? You are not your own; you were bought at a price. Therefore honor God with your bodies."

Is it because you are in pain or tired of feeling sick, lethargic, forgetful, and not anywhere near your best?

> "God is always more interested in why we do something than in what we do. Attitudes count more than achievements."
> — Pastor Warren

Is it because you want to feel healthy and vibrant to live out your purpose, to do the work you love, to be with the people you care about, or to see your grandchildren grow up?

Is it because you want to prevent illnesses that may run in your family, such as diabetes, cancer, heart disease, or Alzheimer's disease?

Write down your motivation — why it is important for you to get healthy — and then look at it daily. We find it most effective if you approach it from two perspectives: To attain benefits, and to avoid negative consequences.

---

### A Mind for the Future

"My greatest motivation is to be healthy in order to model the Lord for my grandchildren and to work with children. For this, I need energy and a clear mind, a ready laugh, and joy in each experience. I notice the responses of others when I look good and feel good; I even notice the nudgings of the Lord more clearly. Perhaps this relates to having a sense of contentment and well-being. I am more loving and more compassionate when my body temple is functioning closer to optimum operating level."

—Mandy Cameron

---

Fifty percent of your brain is dedicated to vision. So it is often helpful to put up what we call "anchor images" to anchor or remind yourself why you want to be healthy. These pictures stimulate motivation. If you want to be healthy to be a great leader of your family, post your favorite picture of your family. If you want to look great, post a picture of yourself when you looked and felt your best. If you want to be healthy to serve out God's purpose, put a picture of yourself doing things that exemplify your purpose.

## BRAIN POWER AND ACTION

A hallmark of intelligence and what separates us from other animals is our ability to think about the consequences of our behavior before acting on impulse.

Effective decisions involve forethought in relation to your goals, which helps you not only to live in the moment, but also to be living ten or even fifty years from now. Boosting your brain power and health will help you avoid troubled situations. Here are seven simple steps to boost your brain and renew your thoughts.

> The most effective people in life think ahead. They know what they want, know what motivates them, keep their thinking honest, and then act in consistent ways over time to achieve their goals.

1. **"Then What?"** The two most powerful words, when it comes to your health, are *then what*. These two small words can literally change your health in a positive way if you keep them at the top of your mind. If I do this, *then what* will happen? If I eat this, *then what* will happen? Does eating the third piece of pizza, skipping the workout, or staying up late help me with any of my goals? Think about the consequences of your behavior before you act.

2. **Get 8 hours of sleep.** Less sleep brings lower overall blood flow to the brain and more bad decisions.

3. **Keep your blood sugar balanced.** Research says that low blood sugar levels are associated with lower overall blood flow to the brain, poor impulse control, irritability, and more bad decisions.[22]

4. **Optimize your omega 3 fatty acid levels.** Low levels of omega 3 fatty acids have been associated with ADHD, depression, and Alzheimer's disease — all brain problems.

5. **Read your purpose-driven goals daily.** Ask yourself, "Is my behavior today lining up with my purpose?"

6. **Practice using your brain.** Self-control is like a muscle. The more you use it, the stronger it gets. Just as good parents help children develop self-control by saying no, strengthen the self-control part of

your own brain by saying no to the things that are not good for you. Over time your brain will make better choices more automatically.

**7. Balance your brain chemistry.** Getting help for problems such as ADHD, anxiety, and depression can help you maintain control over your life.

All of the tools in this chapter work together to help get and keep you focused on the journey toward a healthier life. Making consistently great decisions requires a healthy brain. We gave you a lot to think about. That's the point: We want you to think about your health and become mindful, intentional, and purpose driven. You need a healthy brain and a renewed mind to do that.

### Reflect and Take a Step ...

Be careful what you think, because your thoughts run your life! (See Proverbs 4:23.) Replace any negative thought with one of God's truths. Reflect on his promises and the plans he has for you to prosper. Journal your gratitude daily, and allow God to restore *and* transform your mind.

# Chapter 7

# Friends

*Two are better than one, because they have a good return*
*for their labor (Ecclesiastes 4:9).*

In 2009, the city of Huntington, West Virginia, was plagued with the title of "Fattest City in America" by the Centers for Disease Control (CDC), identifying it as the unhealthiest city in the United States.

For Steve Willis, pastor of First Baptist Church Kenova, near Huntington, the numbers were not just statistics, but lives — and deaths. He was surprised at how many funerals he officiated, especially of people who were dying young of preventable diseases caused by their unhealthy habits.

According to the CDC, Huntington was first (as in *worst*) in the nation in adults who suffered from diabetes (13 percent), first in the prevalence of heart disease (22 percent), and first in the percentage of adults who had no regular form of exercise (31 percent). Nearly half of those over sixty-five had lost all of their natural teeth (first place in that category too)! The city was first in kidney disease, vision problems, and sleeping disorders. Whether it was high blood pressure, circulation issues, or the depression that stems from such unhealthy bodies, the area was the worst in every aforementioned category.

While a few other cities came close to those percentages in some areas, no one else encroached on Huntington's incredible 46 percent of adults who were obese (not just overweight). That's nearly half of the adults. It was, as they say in the sporting world, a total blowout.

In those sobering statistics Pastor Willis heard God calling him to a challenging assignment: preach about health to a very unhealthy congregation. Willis says,

> The transformation began with a declaration of the truth that taking care of our bodies is an act of worship. Nearly half of our congregation struggled with obesity, so [addressing this issue head-on] was one of the most difficult [sermons] I have ever delivered. But nearly a third of our congregation made a public commitment to lose at least forty pounds.

Pastor Willis was delighted at both their response and the life change that occurred.

> I wasn't ready for such a large mass of people (pun intended), but thanks to people like Elizabeth Bailey and my wife, Deanna, we put together a Daniel-like plan for our first set of accountability groups. Each group met weekly for prayer, Bible study, encouragement, and yes, exercise.

Willis believes those groups were the secret weapon in battling the obesity epidemic in the Huntington area.

When you have friends to go with you on the journey toward better health, you are more likely to succeed. Life change happens in small groups. "By creating a culture of both love and accountability, our church has seen many people revolutionize their lives, not only in the physical realm, but in their spiritual and mental lives as well," Willis says.

Willis wrote a book, *Winning the Food Fight,*[1] about the experience of transforming his church, his community, even his own family. These days Huntington is no longer "number one." The city was happy to relinquish its championship status — and in fact worked hard to do so. The statistics have changed because people came together to help each other be healthier. Willis adds,

> Starting with the members of our church, we teamed up with other like-minded groups who cared about our city's health. By implementing the principles of The Daniel Plan, we are no longer

number one in any of those statistics. In fact, if the most recent studies are correct, Huntington has begun to reverse the obesity trend.

Four years later, the church has traded unhealthy habits for healthy ones, from what is served at church potluck dinners to the snacks in the children's department. One church member even donated an acre of land for a community garden.

Most recently the church began educating the children in its preschool about the difference between real food and the processed fake foods that are typically marketed toward children. Willis reports,

These kids are now going home and teaching their parents about the importance of real food and knowing where it comes from. Perhaps the best news is that our children's department has nearly doubled since we have instituted these nutritional changes. We've still got a long way to go, but it continues to amaze me that the more we get physically healthy, the more we seem to be a spiritually healthy body of Christ.

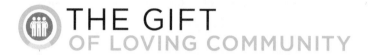

# THE GIFT
## OF LOVING COMMUNITY

**THE STORY OF PASTOR WILLIS'S CONGREGATION** is inspiring. We all love the idea of being healthy — of being our best self emotionally, spiritually, and physically. The Daniel Plan offers you a clear, simple way to be your best, healthiest you.

Improving your health is possible, but doing so requires intention and effort in our daily choices. When we choose to spend time with God, to exercise, to eat healthy food, and to focus our thoughts, we take steps toward our goals in every area of life. That can be hard, especially if we're trying to make changes to existing habits — and even tougher if we try to go it alone.

But the really good news is that God doesn't want you to do it alone. He made you to thrive when you're connected with others. Being engaged in community will improve your health — and not just physically. Friends can improve your emotional and spiritual health.

> "Share each other's troubles and problems, and in this way obey the law of Christ" (Galatians 6:2 NLT).

The opposite is also true: Isolation injures us. Our lack of community can keep us from being the healthiest we can be. In other words, the Friends Essential is the secret sauce for all the other Essentials.

One of the reasons The Daniel Plan has already helped thousands of people to succeed in a healthier lifestyle is the fact that it is done in community. It worked in Huntington, and it will work for you.

## A MEDICAL SOLUTION

Involving your friends is not just a feel-good aspect of The Daniel Plan. Research backs up the concept, showing how crucial we are for each other's healing and success. Much of what currently ails us (and people all over the globe) is preventable, treatable, and very often curable. Even better: the cure is right next to us.

Over the next twenty years, chronic diseases such as high blood pressure, diabetes, and heart disease will cost an estimated $47 trillion to address worldwide.[2] But such diseases are preventable, since their root causes are often being overweight and having a sedentary and unhealthy lifestyle.

For decades, the medical community has tried to solve chronic disease problems with medical solutions — which makes sense, on one level. Medical problems need medical solutions, right? But no part of our life is isolated from another. Our medical travails are tied in part to our lifestyle and our emotions, such as stress and fear. What we eat and how much we move also impact our medical health. So finding a pill or treatment to combat those medical problems doesn't always work. For years, Dr. Hyman wondered why medical science couldn't solve what appeared to be medical problems. Then he read about the work of Dr. Paul Farmer, and Dr. Hyman's perspective changed.

Dr. Farmer was able to successfully treat TB and AIDS — which everyone thought were untreatable in the face of extreme poverty in places like Haiti, Peru, or Rwanda. He realized that the key to treatment was not a new medication but something very simple — to

## Cycling for Food and Health

In Thailand, patients with diabetes take turns pedaling an old bike that is hooked up to a generator to irrigate a community garden.[3] Exercise with teamwork helps them grow their own healthy food. This kind of model of a peer group as the catalyst for health is more effective than conventional medical intervention.

rebuild community and connection in places it had broken down.[4] In other words, friends were the key. Dr. Hyman says,

> Paul's genius was his insight that the key to solving insoluble health care problems was each other — people helping people. Paul's genius was the idea of accompanying each other to health, helping each other build back their communities with clean water, food, going to each other's houses to make sure their sick neighbor knew how and knew when to take their medication.

Our social circles influence our health even more than our DNA. We are more likely to be overweight if our friends are, even if our parents are not. At the same time, we are more likely to exercise and eat healthy food, to not smoke or overeat, if our friends also practice healthy habits. If they're sick, we're more likely to be sick. If our friends have healthy habits, then we probably will.

> Community has the power to change our overall health more than any doctor or clinic.

This means your friends and family may determine how successful you are with The Daniel Plan. If they're healthy, you're more likely to be healthy. If they are focused on their goals with a positive attitude, you will be too. If they are living their faith, you will have built-in support.

In a study published in the *New England Journal of Medicine*, researchers found that one of the strongest associations in the spread of obesity are the people you spent time with. Subjects who had a friend who was obese had a 57 percent chance of also being obese. If the two individuals identified each other as being strong friends, the figure shot up to 171 percent. And this relationship held even if the subjects didn't live in the same area. Sibling relationships also proved important. Having an obese sibling was related to a 40 percent increase in the chance of obesity.[5]

In one of the longest longevity studies ever done, researchers found that health habits are contagious.[6] For example, if you spend time with people who exercise, you are more likely to exercise. If you spend time with people who eat healthy, you are more likely to eat in a healthful way. The group you associate with often determines the type of person you become.

This doesn't mean you have to get rid of all your unhealthy family and friends. Rather, be the leader and model a new way of living.

You are not just receiving influence; you are an influencer as well. If you develop and keep healthy habits, your friends and family are more likely to develop them. Habits are contagious, which means you can have significant effect on those around you. But that may not happen overnight.

> "To get really healthy, find the healthiest person you can stand and then spend as much time around him or her as possible."
>
> — Dr. Amen

Dr. Amen found that he and his wife, Tana, met with some initial resistance from their large extended family when they first changed their eating habits.

> I have five sisters, a brother, living parents, and twenty-one nieces and nephews. When Tana and I first decided to get really healthy years ago, many in my own family thought it was very odd and even made fun of us. I explained why it was important to us to start feeding our brains and bodies in a healthy way.

Dr. Amen's extended family frequently gathered together for meals, which caused noticeable tension when he and Tana insisted on eating differently than the rest of the family. But the two of them supported each other in their new lifestyle. Dr. Amen says:

> Over time, members of our family started coming to us for help. One of my nephews who had been morbidly obese was one of those who asked us for help and ended up making radical changes. When Tana and I took the lead on health and persisted in the face of criticism and initial protests, everyone benefited.

## LOVE AND HEALTH

Major breakthroughs in recent years have significantly altered the way we as Americans care for our health. While we have known for a while that lifestyle can cause health problems (smoking can cause cancer, lack of exercise or excess weight contributes to heart disease), the idea that the reverse is also true — that lifestyle can reverse health problems — is new.

Dr. Dean Ornish discovered four steps to reverse heart disease:

1. Exercise regularly.
2. Eat a plant-based diet.
3. Reduce your stress.
4. Quit smoking.[7]

However, a number of years after clinically proving the effectiveness of these four lifestyle behaviors, Dr. Ornish was frustrated and perplexed why so few followed his proven four-step plan to reverse heart disease and arterial blockage.

He then embarked on a quest to find the deeper answers about why we don't do the very things that we know are best for our health and well-being. He realized that just knowing what to do is only part of the solution. He ultimately discovered after many years of extensive research that there is something deeper that enhances motivation and significantly enhances our ability to naturally choose healthy behaviors and improve our lives.

This Harvard-trained physician discovered that it is relationships that ultimately impact our motivation to exercise and eat healthy. It is love that transforms our health, fitness, and lives more than anything else. He wrote:

> "So now I am giving you a new commandment: Love each other. Just as I have loved you, you should love each other. Your love for one another will prove to the world that you are my disciples" (John 13:34 – 35 NLT).

Medicine today seems to focus primarily on the physical and mechanistic: drugs and surgery, genes and germs, microbes and molecules. I am not aware of any other factor in medicine — not diet, not smoking, not exercise, not stress, not genetics, not drugs, not surgery — that has a greater impact on our quality of life, incidence of illness, and premature death from all causes than love and intimacy! Love and intimacy are at the root of what makes us sick and what makes us well, what causes sadness and what brings us happiness, what makes us suffer and what leads to healing. If a new drug had the same impact, virtually every doctor in the country would be recommending it for his or her patients.[8]

## LIFE CHANGE

Our experience at Saddleback confirms Dr. Ornish's research. When we introduced The Daniel Plan, more than 15,000 people joined us that first year, eager to find friends who could help them. They worked their way through the curriculum, but each group had its own focus and flavor. There was no doubt: Groups were indeed the "secret sauce" of The Daniel Plan, the piece that made this plan succeed where other diet and exercise plans failed. It shouldn't have surprised us, of course. We believe life change happens in community.

### Set a Fitness Date

Find a workout buddy with similar interests. Think about friends, family members, or members of your church who may have similar interests to you, and give them a call and set a date to plan your fitness together. You can even post your interests on Facebook or Twitter to see who responds. Or work out with a family member. Set a weekly date — before the week begins — with your spouse, child, or parent to participate in a fun fitness activity together.

One group of women not only met to study and pray together, but once a week would also shop together for healthy food. They would go back to one woman's house and cook in bulk, making a big batch of turkey chili or healthy chicken salad. They would divide up the

234 The **Daniel** Plan

food and each take home a few premade meals. They had a great time shopping and cooking together, and the conversations as they did so encouraged them even more.

Other support came more organically as people at an exercise class or a Bible study would talk about healthy lunch ideas or give each other tips on juicing, trade recipes, or just encourage each other.

Another Daniel Plan participant lost 45 pounds and radically changed all of her health habits. As she got healthy, her husband, who weighed 300 pounds, at first was resistant to change. But as he saw his wife's success, he joined her in changing his lifestyle. He eventually lost 75 pounds.

Often, the most loving thing you can do for your spouse is to get healthy yourself. This woman showed her husband, by her brave example, that a better life is possible if you do the right things, which in this case ultimately encouraged her husband and her children to get healthier as well.

### A Pastor's Family

"The fight for good nutrition was never more real to me than when I watched my kindergarten-aged son struggle with adapting to his physician-prescribed, mind-altering drugs.

"Lucas had been having discipline problems in school, would frequently struggle with the ability to focus on tasks at hand, and found himself well below grade level in many academic areas. Though his mother was an elementary school teacher who worked with him incessantly, his test scores remained in the bottom 50th percentile.

"So we did what many parents feel forced to do. We placed him on the ADD/ADHD medications that would keep him calm in school, but seemed to stunt his personality and growth in other areas. For his sake, my wife, Deanna, wanted to make radical changes to our family's diet, but I resisted due to my everlasting longing for pizza, French fries, and syrup-laden ice cream. After months of watching our formerly energetic son become totally lethargic and emotionally disconnected, I relented and told my wife, 'Do what you have to do.'

"She implemented the principles of The Daniel Plan in our home right away. Within just three months, our son was completely changed. He was off his medications, the discipline problems had ceased, and his test scores jumped from C's to A's. The change was nothing short of miraculous.

"If you are in the early stages of making the necessary changes for your family, stay the course and fight the good fight. I won't tell you it was an easy sell to replace all the sugary cereals and junk food with healthier options. At first our older children just chose not to eat as much and leave some food on their plates. Eventually their tastes changed, as did mine, and I can honestly say that now I'd rather have a good dish of grilled vegetables than a greasy hamburger any day!

"The good news is that today our teenage daughter is all about cooking healthy food for our family. She recently attended a summer camp, and of all the fun free-time activities, she signed up for the healthy cooking class.

"As for Lucas, the one who once struggled behaviorally and academically, years later he remains an A student in math and consistently scores above the 90th percentile in nearly every category.

"As a pastor and father, I have to wonder: *How many other children are in the same boat as my son? How many other children have the ability to be top mathematicians, scientists, poets, musicians, or athletes, but are being robbed of those capabilities due to an unhealthy diet?* This is more than a health issue; it is a social justice issue. Millions of our children are not reaching their God-given potential because we, as adults, won't take the steps necessary to get them the nutrition they need. For the church, this problem has to be seen as a moral issue. For the sake of our children and our nation's future, we have to do better."

—Pastor Steve Willis

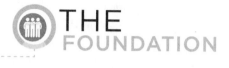

# THE FOUNDATION

**ONE DAY JESUS** was having a lively debate with a bunch of religious leaders, people who defined their faith by rule-keeping. They asked him, "Which is the greatest commandment in the Law?" (See Matthew 26:36–40.)

Jesus' answer was radical in that culture, even more than it would be for us today. They were expecting to hear about rules and the law or to stump Jesus by asking him to pick one of hundreds of religious laws. Instead, Jesus pointed them toward grace, contrasting it with the demands of the law. He essentially told them, "It's not about rules at all; it's about relationships. Life is all about love. It's not about accomplishment. It's not about acquisition. It's not about popularity, power, or prestige. It's about love. It's about relationships."

If you want to have lasting change in your life, then you must fill your life with love. That's why The Daniel Plan success depends on having friends to walk beside you — because love is the only thing that can change the unchangeable. It's the most powerful force in the world. Love invigorates, revitalizes, and renews.

> You can summarize all of life in two sentences: "Love God with all your heart, and love your neighbor as yourself" (see Matthew 22:37, 39).

Love is the most irresistible force in the universe because God is love. And that love is available and accessible to every human being. We don't need to earn it, only embrace it. The Bible doesn't say God has love; it says he *is* love. Love is the core of his very nature. God's love heals what cannot otherwise be healed. God's love uplifts. It strengthens.

## BETTER TOGETHER

There's a wonderful word in the original language of the New Testament that is used to describe the community of the early church: *koinonia*. It is most often translated *fellowship*, a word we sometimes tend to use as a synonym for socializing, perhaps with our church friends.

But *koinonia* means far more than mere socializing or even gathering in a small group. It means love, intimacy, and joyful participation, deep communion with one another — putting others' needs before your own. It's a radical level of friendship and community, similar to that of the early church, described in Acts 2:42 – 47 and elsewhere. It implies a deep commitment, not out of obligation, but out of genuine and joyful love for one another.

God's vision for you is that you would experience *koinonia*.

### Set the Pace for Someone Else

"Leading up to her third marathon, my wife had a simple plan: find her pacer and stay close to him no matter what. Most marathon organizations provide the runners with all sorts of tools and techniques to help them through the grueling course — perhaps most notably, pacers.

"A pacer is a man or woman capable of finishing the race at an exact time. Kevin ran through the finish line at 3:35 — just what he was asked to do. Now, Kevin didn't know who was counting on his pace. All he knew was that someone would be relying on his experience, strength, and endurance to help him or her along their way toward the goal.

"In our daily pursuit of spiritual and physical stewardship, we all need pacesetters: People whom God places in our lives to help us stay the course. Not only that, but God may, in fact, bless us with the privilege of being that for someone else. Like Kevin, we may or may not know who, but someone is depending on us to know the way and show the way."

— Jimmy Pena, exercise physiologist and founder of Prayfit.com

"We are many parts of one body, and we all belong to each other" (Romans 12:5 NLT). God designed us to grow spiritually within a supportive community. The same is true if we want to grow healthier.

### BAN LONELINESS

Researchers tell us that lack of relationship significantly affects our physical and mental health in several ways.[9] When we are lonely, it can cause us to lose focus, struggle in our faith, give up on our fitness goals, and even miss out on fellowship around a food table.

Feelings of loneliness and being disconnected from community can ...

- Increase the likelihood of engaging in unhealthy, self-destructive coping behaviors such as being inactive, smoking, drinking in excess, and overeating.

- Decrease the likelihood that we will make healthy lifestyle choices that are life enhancing, such as exercising, goal-setting, spending time with friends, reading our Bible, or praying.

- Increase the likelihood of premature disease and death from all causes by 200 – 500 percent!

- Keep us from fully experiencing the joy of everyday life.[10]

### Find a Club

Join a walking, jogging, or hiking group. If walking or running is your gig, check out all the resources in your community related to walking or jogging clubs. A great resource is your local YMCA, Sierra Club, and gyms in your area. Some restaurants even host weekly running clubs. Usually fitness facilities in your area will offer free walking and/or jogging clubs. If you can't find any in your area, think about starting your own.

However, when we support each other, we increase one another's potential in every area of life. In fact, the word *support* carries the idea of strengthening one another — to help one another become more capable of facing the challenges of living for Christ and the challenges of health. As Philippians 1:30 tells us, "We are in this fight together" (NLT).

When you connect with a loving community of friends, you will be better able to cope with things like fatigue, fear, frustration, and failure. You will be better able to handle depression and despair and, most important, not have to walk through them alone.

## A WAKE-UP CALL

A member at Saddleback, Debra Miller, appeared to be "fine." No one knew the pain she was hiding. She needed sleeping pills at night, excess caffeine during the day, and pain pills to help her manage back pain. She would get out of breath climbing stairs, but figured that was what happened to everyone in their forties. Yet, being ever the enthusiastic volunteer, she decided to lead a Daniel Plan group. She was not overweight, but even so, as she changed her eating habits, she began to feel a bit better. Still, she knew something wasn't right. "I still felt like I was dying inside, and I still hadn't stopped the medications," she admits.

She finally got a blood test, which revealed how sick she really was: She was profoundly anemic and had bleeding ulcers. The doctors sent her directly to the emergency room for a blood transfusion.

That emergency room visit was a wake-up call, which inspired her to get serious about her Daniel Plan group — which has been an integral part of staying healthy long-term. She decided she wouldn't lead alone. So she and her friend Claudia became co-leaders. Their group took several immediate actions, such as changing the snacks they served at group from cookies and cakes to fruit, vegetables, and nuts. Beyond dietary changes, they cooked together, hiked together, and supported each other.

"To do something alone is really difficult," Debra says. "We are all in it together, because together we are better, all the way around."

## COMMITMENT REQUIRED

Staying in honest, deep relationships is not always easy. It requires commitment. But the flip side is a wonderful gift: When you commit to a few friends or a small group, the people in that group will also commit to you to help you make real and lasting changes. The apostle Paul said, "Your faith will help me, and my faith will help you" (Romans 1:12 NCV).

Commitment is countercultural, and for some of us, it is counterintuitive. We don't want obligations. But commitment is what makes a small group successful because the group members know that they can depend on one another through good and bad times.

If we pretend that everything is fine and we have no real burdens, we will feel lonely and isolated. It's when we're open about our burdens (our weaknesses and struggles) that we find healing and comfort. We find that we are better able to focus and stay mentally and emotionally healthy. We find we are not alone in our struggles to stay on track with our goals. We breathe a sigh of relief, because the doubts and temptations that try to get us off track in our faith are not unique. Others face the same struggles.

"Encourage one another and build each other up" (1 Thessalonians 5:11).

The Bible says openness is a significant step toward healing and wholeness: "Make this your common practice: Confess your sins [faults] to each other and pray for each other so that you can live together whole and healed" (James 5:16 MSG).

We must be brave enough to be authentic — to admit our issues and accept the weaknesses of others. We need to create a community where every member feels accepted and is not afraid to ask for help.

The Bible says, "Therefore, as God's chosen people, holy and dearly loved, clothe yourselves with compassion, kindness, humility, gentleness and patience" (Colossians 3:12). Nowhere in that list does it say to give advice or offer quick, cosmetic help. Rather, it points us to understand and be gentle with the pain of others.

While every group is unique, we support each other by doing the following:

**1. Love each other.** Treat each other with humbleness and patience, no matter where each of you is on the journey. Love accepts us where we're at, but expects us to grow. And love doesn't just mean warm feelings; sometimes it means bringing a hot meal or helping someone with tasks they couldn't do alone.

**2. Listen to each other.** Admit your weaknesses and struggles, your progress and successes. Then listen to your friends as they share the same. Listening means fully engaging, noticing not just verbal, but nonverbal, clues about how someone feels. It is not merely waiting for your turn to talk.

The fellowship of suffering is the deepest, most intense level of fellowship. It's where we enter into each other's pain and grief and carry each other's burdens. It is during times of deep crisis, grief, and doubt that we need each other most. When circumstances crush us to the point that our faith falters, that's when we really need committed and sympathetic friends. We need a small group of friends to have faith in God for us and to pull us through. "If one part suffers, every part suffers with it; if one part is honored, every part rejoices with it"

### Ease the Challenge

Working out with a friend can actually make exercise more effective and less difficult. Researchers from Oxford University discovered that when individuals exercise together they release more "happy hormones" (endorphins) than when they work out alone. Researchers also found that working out in a group decreased feelings of pain and discomfort during exercise.[11]

(1 Corinthians 12:26). In a small group, the body of Christ is real and tangible, even when God seems distant.

**3. Learn from each other.** Share what works and what doesn't. Tell each other about what you have tried in faith, food, fitness, and focus. Talk about what you're learning. You can learn from anyone, so don't assume that someone younger or less experienced can't teach you something.

**4. Liberate each other by showing each other grace.** Increase your encouragement and support when others make mistakes or hit a rut on their journey. When people know they're loved when they face setbacks, your group becomes a safe place where people feel free.

Someone in your group may be wondering, "Am I strange for feeling this way? Am I goofy? Am I mixed up?" You can encourage and affirm that person when you say, "No, you're not weird. You're just acting like the rest of us. We've all been there." Or "I understand what you're going through, and what you feel is neither strange nor crazy."

## My Post-College Team

"As a collegiate athlete, I loved to work out with my team. After graduation, I recruited a group of my old football buddies and friends to meet on a regular basis at the gym. Every morning I'd meet my friends, and we'd get a great workout together: pushing, spotting, encouraging, just like the old days. We did this for years, and our fitness levels were nearly as good as when we were in our playing days.

"Eventually my workout friends and I got married, had kids, and moved away. I found my fitness levels slowly eroding. I still exercised but now by myself.

"I became determined to find another group of like-minded friends to support my fitness — and it was one of the best moves I ever made. We discovered we all have a love for mountain biking. Now we meet every Friday morning and ride

Take a step to create community or deepen the one you already have with family, friends, neighbors, or work associates.

## THE KEY IS FRIENDSHIPS

Solange Montoya, Joan England, Heidi Jacobsen, Wendy Lopez, and April O'Neil were part of a small group that went through The Daniel Plan together, and they definitely found that accountability and encouragement in their group.

Wendy had tried The Daniel Plan on her own, but without friends, she says, "I wasn't able to complete it. I just kind of gave up. This time around, I think, for me the key point was the friendships."

Her friends agree. To make sure they were faithful about attending exercise class, they would attend together and text each other reminders.

Solange says, "I'd be home and I'd be trying to come up with every excuse in the book why I shouldn't go to exercise class. Then my phone

together, getting a long great workout, enjoying the outdoors, and usually spending an additional bit of time grabbing a cup of coffee or breakfast and sharing life together.

"I also discovered four additional blessings in recruiting my new team of fitness buddies. My wife, my daughter, and our two dogs are now on my team. My wife loves to walk and hike —almost as much as our dogs do—so we faithfully walk at least once a day, sometimes twice. This gives my wife and me an opportunity to talk, laugh, and pray together.

"I also work out with my daughter, who is a high school soccer player. We run stairs and perform a boot camp–style weight-training program three times a week. Working out with her challenges me to push myself to keep up with her sixteen-year-old fitness level. I always leave exhausted, but invigorated and so thankful for the time I have with my daughter."

—Exercise Physiologist Foy

would ring, and it'd be Wendy, letting me know she'd meet me at class. Okay, she's waiting for me. I need to go, and if I didn't get that text, it would be so much easier for me to just sit on the couch and not go." The accountability helped both of them, because the person sending the text realized that meant she had to show up as well!

Accountability also helped the group with Focus, Faith, and Food Essentials. Wendy said,

> Being able to have someone pray for you when you're feeling at your lowest, when you're ready to pull in somewhere and grab a cheeseburger, and you know that you can text and say, "Hey, pray for me. Tell me to stop and turn around." That was huge for me. I've tried other diets where I would lose weight in ten days. But this is a life change. It's forever. You learn how to change your eating habits and your friendships.

Whether you are trying to move forward with your mental health (focus), grow spiritually (faith), make better choices when it comes to what you eat (food), or stay committed to an exercise program (fitness), community gives you the support people need. Knowing you're not alone, that others are cheering you on, keeps you motivated. Giving that same support to others gives you joy and a sense of purpose.

## CREATING COMMUNITY

So how can you find that life-changing community that is so important to success on The Daniel Plan? It's not hard, but you do have to seek it out. A great place to start looking, of course, is your church. You're likely to find other people you already know who want to embrace the Faith Essential, which is such an integral part of lifelong health.

The Daniel Plan is flexible. Each group can do what works for them. There's no "wrong" way to have a Daniel Plan group; any step you take is a good one. Perhaps you volunteer in a ministry at your church — would some of your fellow volunteers want to be in a group with you? Or maybe you are already in a small group or a Bible study — would they want to go through The Daniel Plan together?

But don't limit your quest for community to just your church. In fact, often we connect around a shared interest: we have golfing buddies, a book club, a moms group, co-workers. Parents who have children of similar ages will build friendships that start on the sidelines of kids' soccer games or as they volunteer in their children's school.

Why not also find others online? Join an online virtual group. Did you know that you can even experience the expertise, training, motivation, and instruction of a "real time" fitness instructor via your home or office computer? All you will need is a web cam. For convenience, simplicity, and cost, this type of group allows you to connect virtually, but in the comfort and privacy of your own home or office.

Begin by asking God to bring the right people together. Trust that he will lead you as you seek out community. But don't just sit back and wait for the phone to ring. Earnestly begin to look for like-minded friends who might join you on the journey to a healthier you. Be bold in inviting others, keep your eyes open, even in unexpected places. For example:

- Are the people you work with interested in getting more fit and healthy? You might invite some of your co-workers to meet over lunch once a week as a Daniel Plan group. You could even eat together regularly (encouraging one another to make healthy choices), use your lunch hour to walk, or meet at the gym before or after work.

- Perhaps you have a few neighbors who would want to go through this book or *The Daniel Plan, A DVD Study and Study Guide* with you. If you are in a neighborhood book club or Bunco group, perhaps that group of friends might be interested in learning how to live a healthier lifestyle.

- Are you in a sports league such as a bowling or softball league? Why not build on the community you already have around physical activity, and be intentional about the other Essentials in The Daniel Plan?

- If you have young children, get to know the parents of their classmates at school or the neighbor children they play with.

You might even want to do a "family-style" Daniel Plan group, where you gather for a healthy meal and talk about how to build habits of a healthy lifestyle with your kids.

• Find eight (or so) people whom you would love to get to know better or deepen your relationship with. Invite them to start a dinner (or breakfast or weekend lunch) club. Meet for a healthy meal once or twice a month. Rotate from house to house. Schedule the get-togethers as potlucks, and challenge everyone to choose healthy, nutritious recipes to share. At each dinner, plan to talk about food, health, or community. Tell success stories and open up about your challenges. You will leave nourished.

## A BOND THAT HEALS

There is power in community, so just keep looking for friends to join you on your way to a healthier life. Don't give up on it; reach out to others you think might be lonely or needing inspiration. Ecclesiastes 4:9 – 12 reminds us:

Two are better than one, because they have a good return for their labor: If either of them falls down, one can help the other up. But pity anyone who falls and has no one to help them up. Also, if two lie down together, they will keep warm. But how can one keep warm alone? Though one may be overpowered, two can defend themselves. A cord of three strands is not quickly broken.

That cord of three strands is referring to you, God, and the other person. It ties together the Faith and Friends Essentials — the two components that make The Daniel Plan unique from any other health plan. Having God and friends with you as you make changes in your food, fitness, and focus habits is what makes all the difference.

Invite some friends to do The Daniel Plan, A DVD Study and Study Guide together. Go to danielplan.com to register your group and get started.

Of course, it is quite possible for you to do The Daniel Plan alone — for a short time. But if you want to sustain a healthy lifestyle for the long-term, and if you want to have fun doing it as well, grab a few friends.

Community, when you embrace it, doesn't just help you succeed in your goals. It can bring you joy. Through deep relationships with others, you get to live in the love that God wants to give you. When you are surrounded by others who are just as committed to loving their neighbor as you are, then guess what: You're the recipient of that love as well as a giver of it.

As 1 John 4:12 says, "No one has ever seen God; but if we love one another, God lives in us and his love is made complete in us."

### Reflect and Take a Step ...

Don't try to do The Daniel Plan by yourself. Get a buddy or get a few friends together. We want you to experience how friendship makes all the difference in getting healthy — in body, mind, and spirit.

# Chapter 8

# Living the Lifestyle

*Dear friend, I pray that you may enjoy good health and that all may go well with you, even as your soul is getting along well (3 John 2).*

Now that you have read about the five Essentials from Pastor Warren, the doctors, and the fitness expert, perhaps you are wondering if this plan can really work for you. You may be frustrated that other programs haven't worked in the past. Regardless of your starting point, there is great hope for change. Thousands of people across the world have experienced success, enjoying a new way of healthy living.

Dee Eastman is one of those people. Although her journey is scattered with highs and lows — times of great joy and moments of tremendous grief — Dee has applied the practical principles of the five Essentials. She has created new patterns that are lasting, ways of responding to life that reduce stress rather than create it. The Daniel Plan has become her daily practice, and we are confident it can be for you as well.

Life holds challenges for everyone, and Dee's journey has been no different. Her first daughter was born with severe genetic abnormalities and endured several surgeries. But after four short months her baby passed away. In an instant, hopes and dreams of a family were stolen. Dee struggled to understand why God allowed this loss in her life.

Despite tremendous grief and unanswered questions, Dee and her husband moved forward with the dream of having a family. Within a year came a healthy son, and two years after that a healthy daughter.

Then, shortly after, the surprise of a lifetime knocked on their door. Dee was pregnant with identical triplet girls!

Spinning with joy over the news, they had no idea how they would juggle five kids under the age of five. The pregnancy was complicated, and the girls were born early at twenty-eight weeks. Dee learned that two of the triplets had cerebral palsy, and the doctors said one daughter may never walk.

In the years ahead, striving to find a new normal, Dee tried to adjust to the girls' medical issues and the growing needs of her family. But with her still carrying so much grief over the loss and too much to juggle, her health started to suffer. The emotional stress felt overwhelming. Sinking into depression, she developed irritable bowel syndrome (IBS). The physical stress was mounting.

Dee turned to a friend, and that's when the healing began. She experienced firsthand the power of friendship. The Bible talks about this in Matthew 18:20: "For where two or three gather in my name, there am I with them."

That friendship led her to a small group that encouraged her to honestly share her struggles. Adopting the Friends Essential while entering into authentic community became Dee's first step. "I had to learn how to receive, rather than always being a giver. I had to learn how to talk about the difficult things in my life, instead of keeping them hidden." This transformational concept is something that Pastor Rick frequently teaches: We are only as sick as our secrets. To get healthy, we need to share our struggles and be willing to receive help.

Dee's community moved her forward:

> I had hidden my anger and disappointment for all the difficulties God had allowed in my life, but I decided to open up and begin working through my feelings. I realized that I had put God in a tiny box and that the box needed to be blown up. I needed to embrace the mystery of who he is and trust him, even though some of my questions weren't answered. I made the decision to refocus on him, sit still before him, and meditate on his promises. I have learned to live with intention, to notice that in the midst of stress and strain, God can still be in the center.

One way Dee worked on this was to purposely reflect on the goodness in her life. She kept a journal in which she poured out her feelings and ultimately focused on gratefulness, even as life threw curve balls her way. "This has become a moment by moment choice for me, and it comes down to how I manage my thoughts throughout each and every day. Proverbs 4:23 says, 'Be careful what you think, because your thoughts run your life' [NCV]."

With help from a functional medicine doctor, a new eating plan, and a desire to move and regain physical strength, Dee continued making progress. Step by step with practical advice, her physical, spiritual, and emotional health started to improve. Her depression lifted, and within a few months all the IBS symptoms vanished for good.

One healthy step led to another. Dee got out to walk, and she eventually ran, approaching exercise not out of guilt, but because of the healing effect it had on her body. She then ran a 5K, later a 10K, and eventually a marathon. Today she continues to discover all types of movement she enjoys.

Dee's experience is ultimately what made her say yes when Pastor Rick invited her to be the director of The Daniel Plan. The foundational principles in The Daniel Plan have radically impacted her life for many years now. And in her role as director Dee has witnessed people from all walks of life, young and old, embracing the five Essentials to become healthy and strong. It is these stories of transformed lives and the solid principles of the lifestyle that provide a firm foundation for your growth and the ongoing inspiration for your success to be built on.

> Set up your health profile and get more expert advice — go to *danielplan.com* now.

## START WITH ONE THING

One of the most reassuring things about The Daniel Plan is the fact that it is tested and true. Once you decide to take your first step, your journey has begun. After you experience the benefits of your first health choice, change becomes easier.

Many began by simply trying a new health habit, just one small thing. They decided to start the day with breakfast, or add more veggies to their meals, or take a brisk walk each day, or invite a friend to work out. Small steps, yes. But we began to see surprising life change. Simple changes started to add up. Small steps took them closer to their big dreams.

Dr. Oz recommended that we nudge people in the right direction, and that became our goal. We were astonished by the transformation that occurred right before our eyes. Many started to drop a few pounds. Encouraged by their own progress and by the friends who came alongside them, they continued to make healthier choices. Within the first couple of months, those small changes snowballed into big ones; we saw increased energy levels, better sleep, improved mood, and less need for medication.

Dr. Amen has helped patients navigate the change process for nearly thirty years. He says that a gradual approach is the surest way to success. Trying to change everything at once almost inevitably invites disappointment. Don't try to change dozens of unhealthy habits at once. Start with a few vital behaviors — the ones that will have the biggest immediate impact — and go from there.

## Simply Intentional

Think about your morning and evening routines. Do you find yourself working on your laptop or just dashing off a few emails right before bed? Are you completely rushed as you head out the door first thing in the morning? Small changes to your morning and evening routine can be simple, but they can lessen your stress and make you feel more rested. Try something like deciding you won't start working until you've gone for a walk and eaten a healthy breakfast, or won't end your day without prayer and an inspirational reading. Healthy boundaries like those will remind you that you're in control of your choices — and you will then be inspired to make healthier choices throughout the day.

## CHANGE OF MIND

One important truth to remember: God has given you the power to change your life, to set new patterns and reactions. What we have learned is that those changes can be sustained through the Faith Essential.

Your daily choices, with God's limitless power, done with a community of friends, can help you launch each day with intention and purpose. It begins with a shift in perspective: focusing on the good, acknowledging the abundance, and paying attention to who you are and the power within you to choose what is best. This new outlook leads the way to your transformation.

Within every human heart is a desire to improve, grow, and change. It's universal. We might have different reasons for that. What is your motivation or dream?

That big dream, that goal, is one of the reasons you picked up this book: You want to set new patterns and achieve a healthier, more energetic life. And what we have seen over and over on The Daniel Plan is that change is possible. The ability to set new patterns for the long-haul is within your reach. And revisiting your motivation day by day will help you. When you begin to do that, you will be amazed at the strength you find.

Remember how Wendy Lopez's life changed dramatically when she took the simple step of joining a small group? Each woman in the group set two or three small, achievable goals every week. Wendy decided she needed to incorporate regular exercise into her life. She scheduled walks after work, hikes on the weekends, and even made a date with her son at the gym. Her small but key step: She shared her fitness goals with her small group.

This is what makes The Daniel Plan so sustainable. She wasn't alone in her efforts; she had friends who encouraged her as she set and achieved her goals. They would text her to say they were thinking of her and to ask about her walking and hiking.

For the first time in a long time, Wendy felt encouraged. She was hopeful. She began believing she could do this — because she actually was doing it. Taking small steps allowed her to continue and led to big results. Her fitness improved, but so did her confidence and motivation. She began to believe that change was not only possible, but exciting and within reach.

## Long-Haul Progress

Alonso Charles is another person whose small steps led to big results. Weighing in at over 400 pounds, he was sick and tired of being sick and tired. He had lost his confidence. He didn't have the energy to deal with challenges and stress.

Like Wendy, Alonso joined a Daniel Plan small group at Saddleback, and those group members held him accountable to his goals. Since then, he has lost 140 pounds. Now he dedicates the food he eats to God's purposes and doesn't choose the heavier foods that once weighed him down. He knows that change is his choice.

Alonso's focus also improved. He developed a drive to approach his spiritual walk with an openness to what God was doing in his life. His confidence grew, and he began jogging. As his fitness increased, so did his energy, which led to clearer thinking and decision-making. His insecurities and feelings of being inferior were replaced by the hallmark of The Daniel Plan: hope.

Today Alonso participates in sports and still jogs. The asthma he once suffered from has improved dramatically. His journey has fueled new beliefs about God. He finds himself thinking differently: "If God can do this in my life (something I never thought possible), what else can he do?" His small steps have taken him to a place where he anticipates big things from God. He's regained the ability to dream and developed a heart of gratitude. He is a man of God, transformed.

## BRING IN THE GOOD

So often we subscribe to the misguided notion that change requires deprivation — that transformation somehow requires avoiding certain things. We easily focus on what we can't have instead of the abundance of things we can enjoy.

But the truth is, change is much more sustainable when we focus on what we can have, rather than what we can't. For example, we have talked throughout this book about faith. Some people try to be more faithful only following a list of rules and things they need to stay away from. While it's important to honor God's commandments, making corresponding positive choices is what transforms us. Choices to joyfully worship God, to serve and love others, to focus on gratitude, to be kind — these choices lead to replenishing our spirit and growing our faith.

Similarly, when it comes to our physical health, if we focus only on what we can't eat or can't do, we won't be able to sustain the changes we want. But if we focus on bringing in the good and enjoying the abundance of what God has given us, our body, mind, and spirit will become stronger. We will begin to see that things like walking in the morning or reading our Bible and praying are not things we "have to do," but opportunities we "get to take hold of" because they rejuvenate and restore us. We will cultivate a different relationship with food where we see eating healthfully as a way to be kind to ourselves, to lovingly care for our bodies.

This is how the perspective shift begins. We bring in the good not because we "should," but because we long for the benefits a healthy lifestyle brings.

It's really about self-discovery — trying something new and realizing that you actually enjoy it. It can be simpler than we think it is. You will discover that The Daniel Plan lifestyle is bathed in grace, a God-designed way of life that brings energy and passion into your very being.

Bringing in the good is about going to the grocery store or the farmer's market and finding new healthy foods that you enjoy. It's about learning to love foods that actually love you back. Or it might be about getting back on a bike — something you haven't done in a long time — or swimming for the first time since you were a kid and realizing how much fun it is.

As you do these things, your perspective shifts. Instead of telling yourself, "I can't do this; it's too hard," imagine yourself thinking, "Learning and trying new things is a blast, and I'm going to do more of this." Now life becomes an adventure with an unending list of opportunities to explore.

Each of us is in a different place with our health, but the five Essentials open the door to change. Enter in just as you are. Start with one thing, but start. Perhaps you will set a goal in faith to take time in God's Word and be refreshed by his promises. Or you may start by eating more real, whole foods or walking with friends. The best place to start is wherever you are. As you focus on progress, not perfection, you will be equipped to run the race God's set for you.

## RUN YOUR RACE

Prior to the 1968 Olympics in Mexico City, John Stephen Akhwari of Tanzania was just another marathon runner. An Olympic caliber runner, yes. He had won marathons in Africa, running with times under 2½ hours.

He easily qualified for the Olympics. But in Mexico City, Akhwari encountered an obstacle he had never faced before: the altitude, which caused his legs to cramp severely. Still, he kept running. Then, about halfway through the race, he tangled with some other runners and fell. He dislocated his knee, scraped up his leg, and hurt his shoulder as he fell. But he didn't stop. With terrible injuries and cramped muscles slowing him, he labored on and finished the race. He was one of seventy-five people who started the race, and the last of fifty-seven to finish it.

When he finally entered the arena for the final lap, only a couple thousand people were there to see him complete the race. He finished dead last, more than an hour behind the winner. A cheer went up for this brave runner as he circled the now darkened track. Although it seemed that Akhwari had lost the race, everyone who saw him finish knew he was a winner.

In an interview later on, a reporter asked, "Why didn't you quit when you were hurt and bruised, bloody, discouraged? Why didn't you quit?" His answer: "My country did not send me 5,000 miles to start the race; they sent me 5,000 miles to finish the race."[1]

We want to equip you to run the race God has called you to so you can finish it well. Sometimes that means getting up when you fall and continuing forward no matter how slow it may seem.

A crucial step toward running the race well is to remove the things that hold us back. Hebrews 12:1 tells us, "So let us run the race that is before us and never give up. We should remove from our lives anything that would get in the way and the sin that so easily holds us back" (NLT).

You wouldn't run a marathon wearing a winter parka. If you did, you might expend incredible effort — but never finish the race! It seems like a ridiculous example, doesn't it? But so many of us can't figure out why our efforts seem to bring such small results. We get frustrated: "I'm working so hard but feel as if I'm getting nowhere! Why is this so hard?"

It's time to take off the parka. Whatever is slowing you down, leave it behind.

What is the race God intends for you? To answer that, you must first be honest with yourself and ask him to lead the way.

Many of us are losing energy because we have never taken the time to actually think about what is going on in our lives. Dr. Hyman recommends that you simply write a list of everything that gives you energy and everything that drains your energy. Include all persons, places, things, experiences, thoughts, feelings, and foods. What is it that is slowing you down? What brings you joy and helps you thrive? What habits are encouraging you, and what habits are getting in the way?

Then, each week resolve to let go of one thing that drains your energy and add one thing that gives you energy. This is an enlightening exercise to do before determining your goals and steps for the next 40 days.

Energy drains typically fall into one of three categories: unhealthy habits (such as not getting enough sleep, smoking, eating junk food), unhealthy emotions (such as worry, negativity, or anger), or unhealthy relationships (which could be toxic or codependent). Just becoming aware of those is the first step toward change, toward overcoming obstacles. Spending a bit of time in serious self-assessment of your habits is the first step toward living a healthy lifestyle. Then you are ready to put pen to paper and set some initial goals

As you begin to incorporate the goals you long to achieve, are you looking for an endless power source to keep you going? Are you ready to tap into an abundant supply of love and encouragement? The biggest energy source available to each of us is simply the love of God. He ultimately provides the power to change.

He wants you to be filled with his power. He longs to fill you up with his love. It's amazing that he has called us to be his children and that his love for us never ends. He's waiting for us to accept and receive his love. That sounds like a welcoming invitation, doesn't it? Go ahead, open it .

Being close with our Creator, enjoying intimacy with our Father, is foundational to our life here on earth. It is in quiet time with him that you will receive and understand his will for your life.

## REFLECT ON YOUR JOURNEY

The end of this book is not the end of the road. Rather, it is the place where your journey begins. Forty days to a healthier life is the kick-start. In order to keep growing and moving forward, it's important to reflect on our lives. That is why tracking your progress is so important. We have a journal and a mobile app, whichever you prefer. Whatever your choice, we encourage you to record your journey. We can miss out on just how far we have come if we never take time to look back to see the ups and downs in the road and thank God for how far he has brought us.

Reflecting on your journey will help you figure out your next small step. As Pastor Warren often says, you cannot manage what you do not measure. Journaling your progress is practical, and as you make progress, you will be motivated to continue.

Even the setbacks on your journey can help you move forward. If you pay attention and track your progress, a bad day gives you good data. When your progress wavers, pay attention. Don't judge yourself, but learn from your mistakes, as we discussed in chapter 6. What causes setbacks with your food or fitness? Is it when you get too busy? Is it when you don't get enough sleep? Notice patterns, cycles, and reactions — not so you can beat yourself up or feel guilty, but so you have more information from which to make healthier decisions in the future.

> As part of The Daniel Plan, you get a FREE app with recipes, exercises, and social tools to connect with each other. Go to *danielplan.com*.

On The Daniel Plan, there is no condemnation or guilt. We all make mistakes. The goal here is to learn from them and set new patterns in the areas where we need that most. When we track our victories as well as setbacks, we see that God's grace is sufficient, and his love is bigger than any of our weaknesses.

Steven Komanapalli found this to be true. In chapter 2 you read about Steven, who weighed more than 320 pounds and faced several health concerns. Living The Daniel Plan lifestyle, Steven is a transformed man. You already know he lost weight, improved his cholesterol and blood sugar levels, and got off most of his medications.

Steven also began walking and praying with two friends every day. That was a first small step, but it strengthened him to take more steps. Steven focused on casting all anxiety on God, filling his heart and soul with God instead of finding comfort in food. As he reflects on his journey, Steven knows that having friends who can help him is crucial. He feels less hungry but more energetic. He gets out of bed easily in the morning, feeling well rested — something he was unable to do for twenty years.

When Steven reflects on his journey, he is amazed. Tracking his progress regularly brought the needed insight to continue all the changes he is now enjoying. Living the lifestyle has brought him not only health, but also great joy. He now leads a men's group and inspires others to lead healthier lives. Steven says there are no limits to his success, because God is without limits.

## ALL THINGS ARE POSSIBLE

Our greatest desire is that you would embrace The Daniel Plan and the five Essentials, inviting health into every area of your life. Choose to believe that all things are possible with God. Be kind to yourself and trust him. Make God's Word a daily part of your life, and his truths and promises will restore anything that's broken; his love will propel you into a new way of thinking, a healthy approach to each day.

Invite people to join you on this journey. Enjoy the milestones God weaves in as he writes your story. Celebrate your successes. Share your struggles. Make a U-turn when necessary. Reframe failures as guideposts that serve you, not derail you. Get in community and live there, welcoming God's power into every area. This is the secret sauce of The Daniel Plan: getting healthy together, God's way and with God's power.

All five Essentials — faith, food, fitness, focus, and friends — are exactly that: essential. None of them is less important than another. And each supports the others: When you feel weak in one essential, making positive change in the others helps restore your hope. As you move toward making the principles within all five a part of your daily lifestyle, you will have the strength to create change, sustain it, and maintain your motivation. Old refrains get rewritten, new stories are revealed, and life becomes an adventure powered by faith, hope, and love.

## Reflect and Take a Step ...

Living The Daniel Plan lifestyle is one of grace and pace—a way of living that honors God and breathes new life into your body, mind, and spirit. Consider what next steps you would like to take and new goals you would like to set for the journey ahead. We trust that God has so much in store for you as you continue to follow his plans.

# Chapter 9

# Daniel Strong

## 40-DAY FITNESS CHALLENGE

*Start Moving Your Body*

To help you begin your fitness journey we have created the 40-Day Daniel Strong Fitness Challenge with suggested daily exercises — what we like to call your "play of the day" to help you reach your desired fitness goals. Your fitness goal to become Daniel Strong is to exercise six days a week for the next 40 days.

We will show you how easy it can be to move your body over the next 40 days with an easy-to-follow plan. First, you will see a 40-day plan at a glance and then a more detailed, day-by-day, 10-day fitness schedule. This 10-day program will provide you with a template to create your own Daniel Strong Fitness plan, allowing you to exchange exercises you may prefer in place of our suggestions. We have also provided you with varying levels of exercise to choose from, based on your time constraints, goals, interests, and a way to safely make progress. We have also provided you with your next steps after your 40-day Daniel Strong Fitness Challenge has been completed.

## DANIEL STRONG LEVELS

You can select from three levels of exercise, depending on where you are at with fitness right now.

**Daniel Strong 1** is recommended for individuals who are beginning, are restarting, or have time constraints. Recommended movements in this level are designed to help you slowly and safely incorporate exercise into a busy life.

## DANIEL STRONG
### 40-DAY FITNESS PLAN AT A GLANCE

| DAY 1 | DAY 2 | DAY 3 | DAY 4 | DAY 5 | DAY 6 | DAY 7 |
|---|---|---|---|---|---|---|
| Aerobic & Stretch | Strength Training | Aerobic & Stretch | Strength Training | Aerobic & Stretch | Strength Training | Rest |

| DAY 8 | DAY 9 | DAY 10 | DAY 11 | DAY 12 | DAY 13 | DAY 14 |
|---|---|---|---|---|---|---|
| Aerobic & Stretch | Strength Training | Aerobic & Stretch | Strength Training | Aerobic & Stretch | Strength Training | Rest |

| DAY 15 | DAY 16 | DAY 17 | DAY 18 | DAY 19 | DAY 20 | DAY 21 |
|---|---|---|---|---|---|---|
| Aerobic & Stretch | Strength Training | Aerobic & Stretch | Strength Training | Aerobic & Stretch | Strength Training | Rest |

| DAY 22 | DAY 23 | DAY 24 | DAY 25 | DAY 26 | DAY 27 | DAY 28 |
|---|---|---|---|---|---|---|
| Aerobic & Stretch | Strength Training | Aerobic & Stretch | Strength Training | Aerobic & Stretch | Strength Training | Rest |

| DAY 29 | DAY 30 | DAY 31 | DAY 32 | DAY 33 | DAY 34 | DAY 35 |
|---|---|---|---|---|---|---|
| Aerobic & Stretch | Strength Training | Aerobic & Stretch | Strength Training | Aerobic & Stretch | Strength Training | Rest |

| DAY 36 | DAY 37 | DAY 38 | DAY 39 | DAY 40 |
|---|---|---|---|---|
| Aerobic & Stretch | Strength Training | Aerobic & Stretch | Strength Training | Aerobic & Stretch |

**3 Days of Aerobic/Stretch + 3 Days of Strength Training = 6 Days/Wk**

**Daniel Strong 2** is recommended for individuals who have been exercising occasionally or have the ability and desire to spend a little bit more time exercising. Exercises in this level are designed to help you step it up a bit, progressively challenging you to become Daniel Strong.

**Daniel Strong 3** is designed for individuals who are already active and ready for an advanced challenge. The routines found here will take your fitness to another level. At this level, you will find a host of challenging fitness movements and workouts. Level 3 exercises are online; go to *danielplan.com* for more information.

## SUGGESTED EXERCISES

| LEVEL | AEROBIC EXERCISE OR ACTIVE GAMES | STRETCHING OR LOOSENING | STRENGTH TRAINING |
|---|---|---|---|
| DANIEL STRONG 1 | • Walking<br>• Cycling<br>• Stair climbing<br>• Any PLAY from page 172 | • Neck stretches<br>• Shoulder rolls<br>• Alternating toe touches | • Squats<br>• Desk or modified push-ups<br>• Desk or modified plank<br>• Front lunges |
| DANIEL STRONG 2 | • Walking/Jogging<br>• Running<br>• Rope jumping<br>• Competitive basketball<br>• Fitness classes<br>• Any PLAY from page 172 | • Standing forward shoulder reach<br>• Lunge and bend<br>• Walking high kick<br>• Elbow to foot lunge | • Overhead squats or dumbbell squat<br>• Military push-ups<br>• Plank, side plank, & reach unders<br>• Front lunges or dumbbell front lunges<br>• Metabolic movements — fast-paced, high-intensity (e.g., power skipping, jump squats, toe touch jacks) |
| DANIEL STRONG 3 | Visit *danielplan.com* for level 3 exercises | | |

### What level is best for me?

Based upon your interests, goals, time constraints, and current fitness level, select the level that best suits you. No matter which level you choose, always warm up for at least 5 minutes before starting any aerobic or strength exercise. Feel free to exchange the suggested activities found in Levels 1 and 2 on the following pages with exercises or movements listed in chapter 5 that you would enjoy more. For example, if we suggest walking for 20 minutes today and you would rather jog or go on a bike ride, simply replace the activity and perform it for at least 20 minutes. Or if we make a recommendation for strength training and you would rather do something such as a Pilates class, by all means make the switch. Remember, the goal is to help you get moving and stay moving on a daily basis.

### How do I continue to make fitness a regular part of my life?

After you have completed the 40-Day Daniel Strong Fitness Challenge, we encourage you to either move yourself to the next fitness level (e.g., if you are at level 1, advance to level 2; if you are at level 2 now, advance to level 3) or go to *danielplan.com* for more workouts, exercises, and resources. Visit *danielplan.com* or use The Daniel Plan App to find all the encouragement, support, and instruction you need to be Daniel Strong.

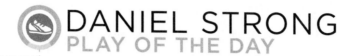

# DANIEL STRONG
## PLAY OF THE DAY

## • DAY 1

Perform the following activities (or exchange with other aerobic activities found on page 172 or on *danielplan.com*).

### LEVEL 1:

**Aerobic:** Go for a 10-to-20-minute brisk walk.

**Stretch:** Standing neck stretches; pray or meditate while doing these. Perform this stretch for 10 to 15 seconds to each side at your desk or when at home throughout your day. (See illustration on page 280.)

### LEVEL 2:

**Aerobic:** Go for a 20-to-30-minute power walk, walk/jog, interval training, or jog.

**Stretch:** Complete

☐ Standing forward shoulder reach

☐ Lunge and bend

☐ Walking high kicks

Perform each stretch or movement (see illustrations on pages 280 – 81) for 10 to 15 seconds each side (or 5 times for each side of your body) before and/or after your aerobic exercise or throughout your day at work or home. Thank God for the blessing of a body that moves.

## DAY 2

Perform the following activities (or exchange with other strength activities found on pages 174 – 75 or at *danielplan.com*).

### LEVEL 1:

Strength: Perform one set of 8 – 10 repetitions
(or as many as you can do):

☐ Squats

☐ Desk or modified push-ups

(See illustrations on page 282.)

### LEVEL 2:

Strength: Perform as many repetitions as you can of each exercise below in 20 seconds. Then rest 10 seconds in between each exercise. Once you have completed all exercises, rest for a full 2 minutes. Complete an additional set for a total of two sets:

☐ Overhead squats: 20 seconds/10 seconds rest

☐ Run in place: 20 seconds/10 seconds rest

☐ Military push-ups: 20 seconds/10 seconds rest

☐ Run in place: 20 seconds/10 seconds rest

☐ Front lunges (alternating sides): 20 seconds/10 seconds rest

☐ Elbow plank: 20 seconds/10 seconds rest

☐ Run in place: 20 seconds/rest

(See illustrations on pages 282 – 83.)

## DAY 3

Perform the following activities (or exchange with other activities found on page 172 or on *danielplan.com*).

### LEVEL 1:

**Aerobic:** Go for a 10-to-20-minute bike ride or walk.

**Stretch:**

- ☐ Standing neck stretches
- ☐ Standing shoulder rolls

Complete each movement for 10 seconds to each side (or 5 to 10 times for each shoulder) at your desk or when at home throughout your day. (See illustration on page 280.) Pray or meditate on Scripture during these loosening movements.

### LEVEL 2:

**Aerobic:** Go for a 20-to-30-minute power walk, walk/jog, interval training, or jog.

**Stretch:**

- ☐ Standing forward shoulder reach
- ☐ Lunge and bend
- ☐ Walking high kicks

Perform each stretch or movement for 10 – 15 seconds on each side (or 5 to 10 times each side) before or after your aerobic exercise or throughout your day at work or home. (See illustrations on pages 280 – 81.) Pray or meditate on Scripture during these loosening movements.

## DAY 4

Perform the following activities (or exchange with other activities found on pages 174–75 or on *danielplan.com*).

### LEVEL 1:

Strength: Perform one set of 8–10 repetitions (or as many as you can do):

☐ Squats

☐ Desk or modified push-ups

☐ Desk or modified planks, hold for 10 seconds

(See illustrations on page 282.)

### LEVEL 2:

Strength: Perform as many repetitions as you can of each exercise below in 20 seconds. Then rest 10 seconds in between each exercise. Once you have completed all exercises, rest for a full 2 minutes. Complete an additional set for a total of two sets.

☐ Overhead squats: 20 seconds/10 seconds rest

☐ Power skipping: 20 seconds/10 seconds rest

☐ Push-ups: 20 seconds/10 seconds rest

☐ Walking lunges: 20 seconds/10 seconds rest

☐ Power skipping: 20 seconds/10 seconds rest

☐ Elbow plank: 20 seconds/10 seconds rest

☐ Power skipping: 20 seconds/rest

(See illustrations on pages 282–84.)

## DAY 5

Perform the following activities (or exchange with other activities found on page 172 or on *danielplan.com*).

### LEVEL 1:

Aerobic: Go for a 10-to-20-minute brisk walk.

Stretch:

☐ Standing shoulder rolls

☐ Standing alternating toe touches

Complete each movement 5 to 10 times (see illustrations on pages 280–81), and thank God for your health as you hold each stretch.

### LEVEL 2:

Aerobic: Go for a 20-to-30-minute power walk, walk/jog, interval training, or jog.

Stretch:

☐ Standing forward shoulder reach

☐ Lunge and bend

☐ Walking high kicks

☐ Elbow to foot lunge

Perform each stretch or movement for 10–15 seconds on each side (or 5 to 10 times each side) before or after your aerobic exercise or throughout your day at work or home. (See illustrations on pages 280–81.) Thank God for your health as you hold each stretch.

## DAY 6

Perform the following activities (or exchange with other activities found on pages 174 – 75 or on *danielplan.com*).

### LEVEL 1:

**Strength:** Perform one set of 8 – 10 repetitions (or as many as you can do):

☐ Squats

☐ Desk or modified push-ups

☐ Desk or modified plank, hold for 10 – 15 seconds

(See illustrations on page 282.)

### LEVEL 2:

**Strength:** Perform as many repetitions as you can of each exercise below in 15 seconds. Then rest 15 seconds in between each exercise. Once you have completed all exercises, rest for a full 2 minutes. Complete an additional set for a total of two sets:

☐ Overhead squats: 20 seconds/10 seconds rest

☐ Toe touches: 20 seconds/10 seconds rest

☐ Push-ups: 20 seconds/10 seconds rest

☐ Toe touches: 20 seconds/10 seconds rest

☐ Walking lunges: 20 seconds/10 seconds rest

☐ Toe touches: 20 seconds/10 seconds rest

☐ Side plank: 20 seconds/10 seconds rest

☐ Toe touches: 15 seconds/rest

(See illustrations on pages 282 – 83.)

## DAY 7                    REST

## DAY 8

Perform the following activities (or exchange with other activities found on page 172 or on *danielplan.com*).

### LEVEL 1:

**Aerobic:** Go for a 15-to-25-minute power walk.

**Stretch:**

☐ Neck stretches

☐ Standing shoulder rolls

☐ Standing alternating toe touches

Perform each exercise for 10 seconds (or 5 to 10 times) at your desk or when at home. (See illustrations on pages 280 – 81.) Concentrate on your breath and the fact that God is the giver of every single breath you take.

### LEVEL 2:

**Aerobic:** Go for a 25-to-35-minute power walk, walk/jog, interval training, or jog.

**Stretch:**

☐ Standing forward shoulder reach

☐ Lunge and bend

☐ High kicks

☐ Elbow to foot lunge

Perform each stretch or movement for 10 – 15 seconds each side (or 5 to 10 times) before or after your aerobic exercise or throughout your day at work or home. (See illustrations on pages 280 – 81.) Concentrate on your breath and the fact that God is the giver of every single breath you take.

## DAY 9

Perform the following activities (or exchange with other activities found on pages 174 – 75 or on *danielplan.com*).

### LEVEL 1:

**Strength:** Perform two sets of 10 – 12 repetitions (or as many as you can do):

☐ Squats

☐ Desk or modified push-ups

☐ Lunges

☐ Desk plank, hold for 20 – 30 seconds

(See illustrations on pages 282 – 83.)

### LEVEL 2:

**Strength:** Perform as many repetitions as you can of each exercise below in 15 seconds. Then rest 15 seconds in between each exercise. Once you have completed all exercises, rest for a full 2 minutes. Complete an additional set for a total of two sets:

☐ Overhead squats: 20 seconds/10 seconds rest

☐ Iso-explosive jump squats: 20 seconds/10 seconds rest

☐ Push-ups: 20 seconds/10 seconds rest

☐ Iso-explosive jump squats: 20 seconds/10 seconds rest

☐ Walking lunges: 20 seconds/10 seconds rest

☐ Iso-explosive jump squats: 20 seconds/10 seconds rest

☐ Side plank reach under: 20 seconds/10 seconds rest

☐ Iso-explosive jump squats: 20 seconds/rest

(See illustrations on pages 282 – 84.)

## DAY 10

Perform the following activities (or exchange with other activities found on page 172 or on *danielplan.com*).

### LEVEL 1:

**Aerobic:** Go for a 15-to-25-minute bike ride or power walk.

**Stretch:**

- ☐ Neck stretches
- ☐ Standing shoulder rolls
- ☐ Alternating toe touches
- ☐ Standing forward shoulder reach

Perform each exercise for 10 seconds (or 5 to 10 times) at your desk or when at home. (See illustrations on pages 280 – 81.) Pray or meditate on Scripture while you hold each stretch.

### LEVEL 2:

**Aerobic:** Go for a 25-to-35-minute power walk, walk/jog, interval training, or jog.

**Stretch:**

- ☐ Standing forward shoulder reach
- ☐ Lunge and bend
- ☐ High kicks
- ☐ Elbow to foot lunge

Perform each movement for 10 – 15 seconds each side (or 5 to 10 times). (See illustrations on pages 280 – 81.) Pray or meditate on Scripture while you hold each stretch.

## DAYS 11 – 20

### LEVEL 1:

Move to Level 2 and perform instructions for Days 1–10.

OR

**Strength:** Stay at Level 1, and increase the number of repetitions for strength training exercises to 12–15 repetitions. (Also increase your plank exercise to 30 seconds.) If you are up to it, complete two total sets of exercises for Days 11, 13, 16, 18, and 20.

**Aerobic:** Stay at Level 1 and increase your aerobic exercise to 20–30 minutes. Perform exercises such as power walking or a light walk/jog for Days 12, 15, 17, and 19.

**Stretch:** Add one additional stretch to your routine for Days 12, 15, 17, and 19.

### LEVEL 2:

Move to Level 3 by visiting *danielplan.com*.

OR

**Strength:** Stay at Level 2, and increase the duration of each strength exercise to 20 seconds. Perform as many repetitions as you can in 20 seconds. Rest 10 seconds in between each exercise. Complete two to three sets for Days 11, 13, 16, 18, and 20, and rest 1.5 to 2 minutes in between sets.

**Aerobic:** Stay at Level 2, and increase your aerobic exercise to 30–40 minutes. Perform exercises such as walk/jog, jogging, rope jumping, running, basketball, or interval training for Days 12, 15, 17, and 19.

**Stretch:** Add one additional stretch to your routine on Days 12, 15, 17, and 19.

## DAYS 21–30

### LEVEL 1:

Move to Level 2 and perform Days 1–10 instructions on Days 21–30.

OR

**Strength:** Stay at Level 1, and increase the number of repetitions for strength training exercises to 15 repetitions (20–30 seconds for plank exercise) and complete two sets of all exercises for Days 23, 25, 27, and 30.

**Aerobic:** Stay at Level 1, and increase your aerobic exercise to 25–35 minutes. Perform exercises such as power walking or a walk/jog for Days 22, 24, 26, and 29.

**Stretch:** Add one additional stretch to your routine for Days 22, 24, 26, and 29.

### LEVEL 2:

Move to Level 3 by visiting *danielplan.com*.

OR

**Strength:** Stay at Level 2, and continue to perform as many repetitions as you can in 20 seconds. Rest 10 seconds in between each exercise. But now complete three to four sets for Days 23, 25, 27, and 30. Also, decrease your rest interval to 1 to 1.5 minutes in between sets.

**Aerobic:** Stay at Level 2, and increase your aerobic exercise to 35–45 minutes. Perform exercises such as walk/jog, jogging, rope jumping, running, basketball, or interval training for Days 22, 24, 26, and 29.

**Stretch:** Add one additional stretch to your routine for Days 22, 24, 26, and 29.

## DAYS 31–40

### LEVEL 1:

Move to Level 2, and perform Days 1–10 instructions on
Days 31–40.

OR

**Strength:** Stay at Level 1, and increase the number of repetitions
for strength training exercises to 15–20 repetitions (30
seconds for plank exercise) and complete two to three sets
of all exercises for Days 32, 34, 37, and 39.

**Aerobic:** Stay at Level 1, and increase your aerobic exercise to
30–45 minutes. Perform exercises such as power walking or
a walk/jog for Days 31, 33, 36, 38, and 40.

**Stretch:** Add one additional stretch to your routine for Days 31, 33,
36, 38, and 40.

### LEVEL 2:

Move to Level 3 by visiting *danielplan.com.*

OR

**Strength:** Stay at Level 2, and perform as many repetitions as
you can in 30 seconds. Rest 10–15 seconds in between each
exercise. But now complete four sets for Days 32, 34, 37, and
39. Also, decrease your rest interval to 1 minute in between
sets.

**Aerobic:** Stay at Level 2, and increase your aerobic exercise to
40–50 minutes. Perform exercises such as walk/jog, jogging,
rope jumping, running, basketball, or interval training for Days
31, 33, 36, 38, and 40.

**Stretch:** Add one additional stretch to your routine for Days 31, 33,
36, 38, and 40.

## Aerobic Activities/Active Games:

1. Walking
2. Stair Climbing
3. Cycling
4. Walk/Jog
5. Running
6. Rope Jumping
7. Basketball/Competitive Sports
8. Fitness Classes
9. Interval Training

Additional Aerobic Activities and Active Games can be found on pages 172 and 173 or at *danielplan.com*

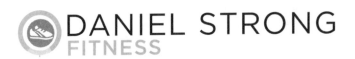
# DANIEL STRONG
## FITNESS

**Neck stretch chin to chest:** Slowly begin to lower your neck down by lowering your chin down to your chest and hold for 10 – 15 seconds.

**Neck stretch ear to shoulder:** Lower your right ear toward your right shoulder. Hold. Lower your left ear toward your left shoulder. Hold.

**Neck Rotation:** Slowly turn your head to the right. Your chin will be close to your right shoulder. Hold. Slowly turn your head to the left. Your chin will be close to your left shoulder. Hold.

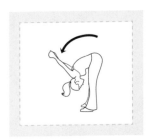

**Standing forward shoulder reach:** Reach your arms behind your back and interlace your fingers. Lift your shoulders up toward your ears, and lift your hands away from your back. Slowly bend forward at the waist, keeping your back flat, not rounded. Continue bending forward, and lift your hands over your head as far forward as comfortable. At a full stretch, you will feel tension in your hamstrings and in your shoulders.

**Shoulder rolls:** Stand with your arms hanging straight down. Shrug both shoulders forward and up. Roll the shoulders back and down. Make big circles while keeping the head straight.

**Alternating toe touches:** Stand with your feet spread as far apart as comfortably possible. Then lean forward toward one leg and try to reach your foot or until you feel a comfortable stretch in your lower back and hamstrings. Now try to touch the other foot with the opposite arm.

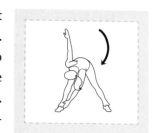

**Lunge and bend:** Stand tall with your arms hanging at your sides. Step forward with your right leg, and lower your body until your right knee is bent at about 90 degrees. As you lunge, reach over your head with your left arm and bend your torso to your right.

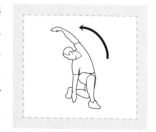

**Walking high kick:** Stand tall with arms hanging at your sides. Keeping your knee straight, kick your right leg up and reach with your left arm out to meet it as you simultaneously take a step forward. (Imagine that you're a British soldier. As soon as your right foot touches the floor, repeat the movement with your left foot and right arm.)

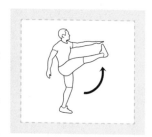

**Elbow to foot lunge:** Brace your core and lunge forward with your right leg. As you lunge, lean forward at your hips and place your left hand on the floor so it's even with your right foot. Place your right elbow next to the instep of your right foot (or as close as you can), and hold. Next, rotate your torso up and toward the right, reaching as high as you comfortably can with your right hand. Repeat with your left leg and left arm.

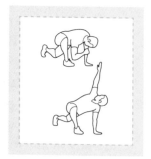

## STRENGTH TRAINING EXERCISES

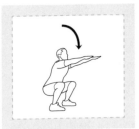

**Squats or overhead squat:** Stand with your feet spread shoulder-width apart. Hold your arms straight out in front of your body at shoulder level.

Your lower back should be naturally arched. Brace your core and hold it that way.

Lower your body as far as you can by pushing your hips back and bending your knees, as if you are sitting down. Pause, then slowly push yourself back to the starting position.

*Tips:* Keep your weight on your heels, not your toes, for the entire movement. Your knees should stay over the centers of your feet as you squat. Your torso should stay as upright as possible. Don't let your lower back round.

For an overhead squat, hold your arms over your head throughout the movement and repetitions.

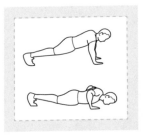

**Push-ups:** Position yourself with your hands slightly wider than your shoulders. Your body should form a straight line from your ankles to your head. Brace your abdominals — as if you were about to be punched in the gut — and maintain that contraction for the duration of this exercise. This helps keep your body rigid and doubles as core training. Lower your body until your chest nearly touches the floor. Tuck your elbows as you lower your body so that your upper arms form a 45-degree angle with your body in the bottom of the movement. Pause at the bottom and then push yourself back up.

For a modified push-up, instead of performing the exercise with your legs straight, bend your knees and cross your ankles behind you. Your body should form a straight line from your head to your knees.

**Plank:** Start to get into a push-up position, but bend your elbows and rest your weight on your forearms instead of on your hands. Your elbows should be directly under your shoulders. Your body should form a straight line from your 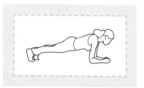 shoulders to your ankles. Brace your core by contracting your abs. Squeeze your glutes. Hold the position.

*Desk or modified:* Perform the plank motion using a push-up position or on elbows, but use a desk to lean on. Or, instead of being on your toes, place both knees on the ground.

**Side plank:** Lie on your left side with your knees straight. Prop up your upper body on your left elbow and forearm. Position your elbow under your shoulder. Brace your core by contracting your abs forcefully as if you were 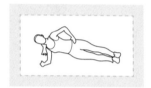 about to be punched in the gut. Raise your hips until your body forms a straight line from your ankles to your shoulders. Your head should stay in line with your body. Hold this position for the prescribed amount of time while breathing deeply.

**Side plank with reach under:** Lift your body into a side plank, and start with your right arm raised straight above you so that it's perpendicular to the floor. Reach under and behind your torso with your right hand, then lift your arm back up to the starting position.

**Lunges:** Stand with your arms by your sides, cross your arms in front of your chest, or place your hands on your hips or behind your ears. Step forward with your right leg and slowly lower your body until your front knee is bent as close to 90 degrees as possible. Pause, then push yourself to the starting position as quickly as you can. Alternate legs after each repetition.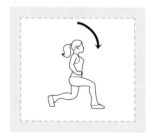

*Walking lunges:* Instead of returning to your starting position, bring your back foot forward and move into a lunge on that leg.

## METABOLIC MOVEMENTS

These create fast-paced, high-intensity aerobic exercises.

**Power skipping:** Raise the right knee up toward the hip while reaching your left arm overhead. Land on the ball of your left foot, and then alternate the skipping motion with the opposite arm and leg.

**Stair sprints:** Run up a set of stairs as fast as you possibly can.

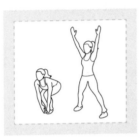

**Toe touch jacks:** Stand with your feet together, arms by your sides. Bend your knees and squat down, reaching your fingertips down to your feet (and if you can, touch your toes). Quickly jump up and open arms and legs, landing in a traditional jumping jack position.

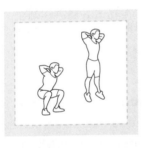

**Iso-explosive squat jumps:** Place your fingers on the back of your head and pull your elbows back so that they're in line with your body. With your feet spread shoulder-width apart, push your hips back, bend your knees, and lower until your upper thighs are parallel to the floor. Your torso should stay as upright as possible. Don't let your lower back round. Keep your weight on your heels, not your toes. Your knees should stay over the centers of your feet during your squat.

Push off the ground so you jump up in the air. Land softly and return to the starting position.

# Chapter 10

# 40-Day Meal Plans
## EAT FOR HEALTH

Based on real, whole ingredients, the 40-day meal plan (and The Daniel Plan Detox) offers meals with a balanced proportion of macronutrients to balance blood sugar, hormone levels, and mood stability and also promote cardiovascular health. Eating frequent, clean, small meals throughout the day will not only help you stay energized, but it will also supercharge your metabolism. This way of eating is the most effective way of losing fat and maintaining healthy muscle mass. You will feel satisfied without that "overstuffed" sensation.

This plan will help you get into the habit of putting together balanced, wholesome nourishment that's easy for your everyday routine. We give you a 10-day chart as your dashboard for planning ahead. You will find that getting meals ready in advance will help you stick with it. So you will use this same chart for the subsequent 30 days, but you can swap meal and snack options for different days to keep your choices fresh. Copy the shopping guide to take to the grocery store for an easier shopping trip.

This meal plan includes a combination of meals that require a recipe (which are on pages 304–31 after the meal plan charts) and meals that require nothing but the description given. Every dish is simple to make with ingredients you can find at any store. Feel free to swap out fruits and vegetables based on the season or your tastes. Explore different spices and herbs to add flavor. Bring your family and friends into the kitchen to partake in the creation of meals. When you follow The Daniel Plan approach, every bite counts that much more.

*Note:* Even though you will find the core meal plan listed first, we encourage everyone to start with The Daniel Plan Detox to see how much better your body can feel. Following the detox plan for a minimum of 10 days may be the best plan for you to use on a regular basis if you have issues with gluten or dairy; you will feel better off them.

## More Recipes

Visit *danielplan.com* for more recipes that use real, whole food for delicious entrees, sides, and snacks. Also, pick up a copy of *The Daniel Plan Cookbook: Healthy Eating for Life* for exclusive recipes by The Daniel Plan signature chefs.

# 40-DAY CORE MEAL PLAN

Meals that require a recipe are in **bold**; you will find the recipes on pages 304–31.

| | DAY 1 | DAY 2 | DAY 3 | DAY 4 | DAY 5 |
|---|---|---|---|---|---|
| BREAKFAST | **Strawberry coco choco shake** | Breakfast muffin: 1 scrambled egg, 2 slices baked nitrate-free turkey bacon or avocado on whole grain or sprouted grain English muffin | **Blueberry, spinach & flax smoothie** | 1 c. rolled or steel cut oatmeal with ½ c. almond milk & ½ c. mixed strawberries and bananas | Breakfast wrap: 1 scrambled egg with ¼ avocado, sliced tomato, basil wrapped in whole grain tortilla |
| SNACK | ⅓ c. **artichoke hummus** with mixed veggie sticks (celery, carrots, cucumber, jicama) | Small apple plus 25 raw almonds | **1 no-bake power bite** | 2 tbsp. **crunchy chickpeas** with 1 oz. hard cheese | Small pear or apple with 1 tablespoon almond butter |
| LUNCH | ½ c. quinoa with steamed broccoli, carrots, cauliflower, & **antioxidant dressing** | Low-sodium, nitrate-free turkey breast wrap with tomato, lettuce, 2 tbsp. **artichoke hummus** | **Veggie lentil & chicken sausage soup** | **Grilled citrus salmon** with **supergreens watermelon salad** | **Grilled citrus chicken wrap** with 2 tbsp. **artichoke hummus,** romaine & ¼ avocado |
| SNACK | 2 tbsp. **crunchy chickpeas** with 1 mozzarella cheese stick | 1 piece low-glycemic fruit plus 25 raw almonds | **Baba ganoush dip** with mixed veggie sticks (celery, carrots, cucumber, jicama) | **1 no-bake power bite** | **Strawberry coco choco shake** |
| DINNER | Open-faced ground beef or turkey burger on ½ whole grain English muffin or bun with spinach, tomato, & 1 tbsp. avocado | **Citrus chicken skewers** with brown rice & **supergreens watermelon salad** | **Grilled citrus salmon** with grilled/baked asparagus and quinoa | **Grilled lamb kofta** and mixed greens salad | **Veggie lentil & chicken sausage soup** with side of quinoa or brown rice |
| HEALTHY TREAT | 1 piece of fruit chopped and sprinkled with cinnamon | **Dark chocolate avocado mousse cup** | **Grapefruit and pomegranate salad with coconut** | **Chocolate and walnut dipped frozen banana pops** | Chopped fruit salad |

## 40-DAY CORE MEAL PLAN cont.

Meals that require a recipe are in **bold**; you will find the recipes on pages 304–31.

| | DAY 6 | DAY 7 | DAY 8 | DAY 9 | DAY 10 |
|---|---|---|---|---|---|
| BREAKFAST | **Supercharged bulgur wheat breakfast bowl** | Breakfast muffin: 1 scrambled egg, 2 slices baked nitrate-free turkey bacon or avocado on whole grain or sprouted grain English muffin | **Mango coconut power smoothie** | 2 hardboiled eggs with mixed fruit cup | 2 hardboiled eggs with mixed fruit cup |
| SNACK | **Berry protein smoothie** | 2 tbsp. nuts and 1 oz. hard cheese | **Creamy carrot dip** with whole grain chips or veggies | 2 tbsp. **dark chocolate trail mix** | **Gluten-free tortilla chips** with ⅓ c. **confetti salsa** |
| LUNCH | **Broccoli fritatta** with mixed greens & antioxidant dressing | **Shrimp curry with snap peas and water chestnuts** | **Crockpot beef and veggie stew** | Grilled fish or chicken with ½ c. quinoa & ½ c. **confetti salsa** | **Crunchy Mediterranean salad with grilled shrimp** |
| SNACK | **Creamy carrot dip** with whole grain chips or veggies | **Dark chocolate trail mix** | Small banana with 1 tbsp. nut butter | **Blueberry, spinach, & flax smoothie** | 1 c. steamed edamame with soy sauce or tamari |
| DINNER | **Crockpot beef and veggie stew** | 2 **grilled fish tacos** with fresh pineapple salsa | **Thai-inspired stir fry with coconut rice** | **Savory oven-fried chicken with cauliflower mash** and baked/grilled asparagus | **Ground turkey/beef and broccoli pasta** |
| HEALTHY TREAT | 1 serving **light pumpkin pie squares** | **Greek yogurt** with **no-sugar-added muesli** | Frozen real fruit popsicles (puree your favorite fruit and freeze) | 1 serving **light pumpkin pie squares** | **Frozen coconut berry dessert** |

| ADDITIONAL BREAKFAST OPTIONS | | |
|---|---|---|
| Mediterranean breakfast: 2 scrambled eggs with ½ c. fresh spinach, 1 tbsp. feta cheese, and 3 chopped kalamata olives | Slice of whole grain toast with 1 tbsp. nut butter and 1 tsp. raw honey with 1 c. fresh melon | ½ c. quinoa with unsweetened coconut milk and 1 tbsp. dried currants |
| 2 scrambled eggs with a corn tortilla, slice of avocado, and 2 tbsp. salsa | 1 whole grain waffle with 1 tbsp. pure maple syrup and 1 turkey sausage | 1 c. plain Greek yogurt with low-sugar granola and blueberries |

| ADDITIONAL LUNCH OPTIONS | | |
|---|---|---|
| **Chicken primavera bowl** | ½ c. brown rice, steamed broccoli and carrots, and diced chicken breast | Open-faced ground bison/ buffalo burger with sliced tomato, spinach, and avocado |
| 1 c. **carrot avocado soup** and a mixed green salad | Mixed green and veggie salad with canned fish and ½ c. mixed fruit | **Herbed fish salad** with mixed greens |

| ADDITIONAL DINNER OPTIONS | | |
|---|---|---|
| **Ground turkey stuffed bell pepper** | **Greek baked cod** | Cucumber, olive, tomato, and red onion salad topped with grilled shrimp, lemon, and olive oil |
| **Whole grain spaghetti alla lucca** | Whole roasted chicken with Brussels sprouts and carrots | Stir-fry eggplant and zucchini with sesame oil and soy sauce, serve over brown rice |

| ADDITIONAL SNACK OPTIONS | | |
|---|---|---|
| **Crunchberry yogurt parfait** | Roasted sweet potato fries | ½ whole grain English muffin with 2 tbsp. cottage cheese and sliced fresh peaches |
| 1 c. whole grain chips with hummus or salsa | 1 c. sliced melon and berries | Whole grain tortilla filled with 3 oz. sliced turkey breast, sprouts, tomato, 1 tbsp. Dijon mustard, and 3 avocado slices |

# SHOPPING LIST
## for the 40-Day Core Meal Plan

Get stocked for success! You can add or modify as needed.

**Important notes:**

1. Compare your shopping list to what's already in your pantry before you go shopping.

2. If the specific size of an item is not listed, you can buy the smallest version. Wherever possible, we indicate how much you will use every five days so you don't end up buying more than you need.

3. Suggested quantities are based on the recipe serving sizes. Entrees generally serve 4; snacks generally serve 1 – 2.

4. * Marks items you will use in Days 1 – 5 and need to repurchase for Days 6 – 10; † indicates a perishable ingredient that is required only for Days 6 – 10.

5. Should you choose to skim the recipes and meals first and swap the items in the plan, you will need to adjust your shopping list accordingly.

### FRESH PRODUCE

- ☐ 4 apples*
- ☐ 2 avocados*
- ☐ 4 bananas*
- ☐ 1 large container blueberries
- ☐ 4 lemons*
- ☐ 2 limes*
- ☐ 2 peaches†
- ☐ 1 pineapple†
- ☐ 1 orange
- ☐ 1 pink grapefruit
- ☐ 1 pomegranate
- ☐ 1 large container strawberries
- ☐ 4 medium tomatoes†
- ☐ Small watermelon or other melon
- ☐ 1 package arugula
- ☐ 1 bunch asparagus*
- ☐ 2 bags (8–9 oz.) of fresh baby spinach, or one small bunch*
- ☐ 2 red bell peppers*
- ☐ 1 head broccoli*
- ☐ 2 heads purple or green cabbage†
- ☐ 1 bag carrots*

* Marks items you will use in Days 1–5 and need to repurchase for Days 6–10
† Indicates an ingredient that is required only for Days 6–10

- ☐ 1 head cauliflower†
- ☐ 1 bag celery*
- ☐ 1 bunch cilantro†
- ☐ 2 cucumbers†
- ☐ 1 eggplant
- ☐ 1 bulb garlic*
- ☐ 1 jalapeno†
- ☐ 1 jicama
- ☐ 2 packages or heads of kale

- ☐ 2 medium onions
- ☐ 2 red onions†
- ☐ 1 bunch parsley*
- ☐ 2 medium red-skinned or purple potatoes or 1 turnip
- ☐ 1 head romaine lettuce*
- ☐ 1 pound snap peas†
- ☐ 1 small bag snow peas or green beans
- ☐ 4–6 zucchini†

## BAKERY/BREADS

- ☐ 1 package taco-sized sprouted or whole grain tortillas
- ☐ 1 package corn tortillas

- ☐ 1 package sprouted whole grain muffins

## MEAT/FISH

- ☐ 2 pounds chicken breasts or cutlets
- ☐ 12 chicken legs†
- ☐ 6 chicken sausages
- ☐ 3–4 pounds chuck roast
- ☐ 1 pound lean ground turkey or beef*

- ☐ 1 pound sliced turkey breast, nitrate-free
- ☐ 3/4 pound halibut or hearty white fish†
- ☐ 2 pounds wild shrimp†
- ☐ 2 pounds wild salmon*
- ☐ 2 cans/packages low-mercury tuna or wild salmon

## EGGS & DAIRY

- ☐ 1 dozen cage-free or organic eggs*
- ☐ 1 small package feta cheese
- ☐ 1 large container nonfat plain Greek yogurt*

- ☐ 1 small package fresh parmesan cheese†
- ☐ 1 package hard, unprocessed cheese

\* Marks items you will use in Days 1–5 and need to repurchase for Days 6–10
† Indicates an ingredient that is required only for Days 6–10

## PASTAS, GRAINS, LEGUMES

- ☐ 1 package brown (preferably jasmine) or black rice
- ☐ 1 package bulgur wheat
- ☐ 1 pound gluten-free pasta (e.g., brown rice pasta)
- ☐ 1 pound lentils
- ☐ 1 container old-fashioned rolled or steel cut oats
- ☐ 1 package quinoa

## FREEZER SECTION

- ☐ 1 package mixed frozen berries
- ☐ 1 package frozen corn
- ☐ 1 package frozen edamame
- ☐ 1 package frozen mango
- ☐ 1 package frozen strawberries

## CANNED FOODS

- ☐ 1 jar unsweetened applesauce
- ☐ 1 can artichokes in water
- ☐ 2 15-oz. cans low-sodium beef broth
- ☐ 1 15-oz. can cannellini, great northern, or black beans
- ☐ 3 cans garbanzo beans/chickpeas
- ☐ 2 qts. low-sodium chicken or vegetable broth
- ☐ 1 jar kalamata or black olives
- ☐ 1 can pumpkin
- ☐ 2 containers fresh salsa or your favorite recipe
- ☐ 1 can chopped tomatoes
- ☐ 1 15-oz. can organic tomato sauce
- ☐ 1 can water chestnuts

## CONDIMENTS/SAUCES

- ☐ 1 bottle unfiltered apple cider vinegar
- ☐ 1 bottle balsamic or red wine vinegar
- ☐ 1 container coconut oil or grape seed oil
- ☐ 1 bottle Dijon mustard
- ☐ 1 bottle extra-virgin olive oil (or cooking spray)
- ☐ 1 jar raw honey
- ☐ 1 small bottle low-sodium soy sauce or tamari
- ☐ 1 small bottle sesame oil
- ☐ 1 small bottle sesame tahini paste

- ☐ 1 small bag stevia or approved natural sweetener
- ☐ 1 can tomato paste
- ☐ 1 jar organic or vegan mayonnaise

## NUTS/SEEDS

- ☐ 1 box unsweetened coconut milk or almond milk*
- ☐ 1 box unsweetened almond milk
- ☐ 1 jar almond or other nut butter
- ☐ 1 bag almond meal/flour
- ☐ 1 bag raw almonds
- ☐ 1 bag slivered almonds
- ☐ 1 package chia seeds
- ☐ 1 bag unsweetened shredded coconut
- ☐ 1 package ground flax meal
- ☐ 1 bag unsalted sunflower seeds
- ☐ 1 bag raw walnuts

## MISCELLANEOUS

- ☐ Dried blueberries
- ☐ 1 container chocolate flavor plant-based protein powder optional
- ☐ 70% cocoa chocolate chips/bar
- ☐ Cornstarch
- ☐ Raisins
- ☐ 1 package organic tempeh (usually in the refrigerator section)
- ☐ 1 container quality plant-based protein powder

## SPICES/HERBS

- ☐ Black pepper
- ☐ Cayenne pepper
- ☐ Chili powder
- ☐ Cumin
- ☐ Curry powder
- ☐ Dill
- ☐ Dry mustard
- ☐ Dried oregano
- ☐ Garlic powder
- ☐ Kosher or sea salt
- ☐ Onion powder
- ☐ Pumpkin pie spice
- ☐ Vanilla extract

* Marks items you will use in Days 1–5 and need to repurchase for Days 6–10

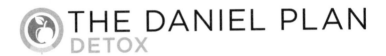

# THE DANIEL PLAN
## DETOX

**THE DANIEL PLAN DETOX** includes the fundamentals laid out in The Daniel Plan. The only difference is that you stop eating anything that could *potentially* trigger health issues. Even if you think you don't have a problem, you might see a big difference. If a horse had been standing on your foot your whole life, then you may not know how bad it feels until he gets off your foot. Most of Dr. Hyman's patients say, "Dr. Hyman, I didn't know I was feeling so bad until I started feeling so good!" That is our wish for all of you.

### *What you will eat:*

- Eat real fresh, whole food.
- Follow The Daniel Plan Detox meal plan chart, or create your own from the real food ingredients.

### *What you will let go of:*

- Stimulants and sedatives: alcohol, caffeine, etc.
- Processed or fast food (get rid of any additives or chemicals)
- Artificial sweeteners of all kinds
- All sugar in any form (see page 108)
- All dairy (milk, yogurt, butter, cheese) 100%, not even a drop
- All gluten (wheat, rye, barley, oats, spelt, kamut) 100%, not even a crumb

## HOW DO I DO THE DANIEL PLAN DETOX?

The Daniel Plan Detox is easier to do in a group or with friends. Find a friend or small group and do it together. You will be enjoying a delicious variety of whole fresh foods and stopping inflammatory or toxic foods. Your body will have a chance to heal, reboot, and reset, allowing you to notice for the first time how good you can really feel. It may seem like a sacrifice, but if you have never done it, you owe it to yourself to learn firsthand how profound healing can come from a few simple dietary changes.

If you are on caffeine, you can slowly cut down by half over the course of a week before you do the detox. That will minimize any caffeine withdrawal headaches. Be sure to drink at least 8 glasses of water a day. Get plenty of sleep, rest, and even naps while your body is healing. Do gentle exercise such as a 30-minute walk a day. Try to cut down on any unnecessary activities or overscheduling; think of this as a time of renewal and restoration. At the end of the 10 (or 40) days, your body will tell you what it needs. If you feel great, just continue eating according to the detox meal plan.

If you want to add back healthy forms of dairy or gluten, then make sure you add one at a time. Start with dairy. Have something a few times a day and notice how you feel. Do you have congestion, bloating, or other symptoms? If you do, then you would mostly likely be better off without it. After three days of eating dairy, add back gluten. Have a piece of bread or some whole grain pasta, and observe carefully. Do you have joint pain, brain fog, headaches, or stomach problems? If gluten makes you sick, or even just sluggish and tired, you want to consider eating gluten free or going on a very low gluten diet. Also, you may try lower gluten grains such as rye or barley or steel cut oats.

Many people have low-grade food sensitivities, and The Daniel Plan Detox is a wonderful way to learn how these two common inflammatory foods affect you.

Adding back caffeine from coffee or tea is also optional. Notice how you feel without the caffeine. You can always have decaf. With that said, however, it is not bad to enjoy your daily cup of joe. Just be sure you don't load it up with lots of sugar or artificial sweeteners. For those who enjoy a drink from time to time, again, it can be part of a healthy lifestyle. Just notice how it makes you feel, how it affects your sleep, energy, and mood. We are all different, and it is key to find the right balance for you.

Fill out the following medical-symptom questionnaire that assesses your overall level of well-being as well as any toxicity or inflammation. Score yourself before and after The Daniel Plan Detox, or at the end of the 40 days. You will be surprised by how much you can heal in such a short time.

## THE TOXICITY AND SYMPTOM SCREENING QUESTIONNAIRE

This questionnaire identifies symptoms that help to identify the underlying causes of illness and helps you track your progress over time. Rate each of the following symptoms based on your health over the past 30 days. If you are filling out this questionnaire after the first two days of detox, record your symptoms for the last 48 hours ONLY.

### POINT SCALE

0 = Never or almost never have the symptom
1 = Occasionally have it, effect is not severe
2 = Occasionally have it, effect is severe
3 = Frequently have it, effect is not severe
4 = Frequently have it, effect is severe

### DIGESTIVE TRACT

_____ Nausea or vomiting

_____ Diarrhea

_____ Constipation

_____ Bloated feeling

_____ Belching, or passing gas

_____ Heartburn

_____ Intestinal/stomach pain

TOTAL _____

### EARS

_____ Itchy ears

_____ Earaches, ear infections

_____ Drainage from ear

_____ Ringing in ears, hearing loss

TOTAL _____

## EMOTIONS

_____ Mood swings

_____ Anxiety, fear, or nervousness

_____ Anger, irritability, or aggressiveness

_____ Depression

TOTAL _____

## ENERGY/ACTIVITY

_____ Fatigue, sluggishness

_____ Apathy, lethargy

_____ Hyperactivity

_____ Restlessness

TOTAL _____

## EYES

_____ Watery or itchy eyes

_____ Swollen, reddened, or sticky eyelids

_____ Bags or dark circles under eyes

_____ Blurred or tunnel vision (does not include near- or far-sightedness)

TOTAL _____

## HEAD

_____ Headaches

_____ Faintness

_____ Dizziness

_____ Insomnia

TOTAL _____

## HEART

_____ Irregular or skipped heartbeat

_____ Rapid or pounding heartbeat

_____ Chest pain

TOTAL _____

## JOINTS/MUSCLES

_____ Pain or aches in joints

_____ Arthritis

_____ Stiffness or limitation of movement

_____ Pain or aching in muscles

_____ Feeling of weakness or tiredness

TOTAL _____

## LUNGS

_____ Chest congestion

_____ Asthma, bronchitis

_____ Shortness of breath

_____ Difficult breathing

TOTAL _____

## MIND

_____ Poor memory

_____ Confusion, poor comprehension

_____ Poor concentration

_____ Poor physical coordination

_____ Difficulty in making decisions

_____ Stuttering or stammering

_____ Slurred speech

_____ Learning disabilities

TOTAL _____

## MOUTH/THROAT

_____ Chronic coughing

_____ Gagging, frequent need to clear throat

_____ Sore throat, hoarseness, loss of voice

_____ Swollen or discolored tongue, gum, lips

_____ Canker sores

TOTAL _____

### NOSE

_____ Stuffy nose

_____ Sinus problems

_____ Hay fever

_____ Sneezing attacks

_____ Excessive mucus formation

TOTAL _____

### SKIN

_____ Acne

_____ Hives, rashes, or dry skin

_____ Hair loss

_____ Flushing or hot flushes

_____ Excessive sweating

TOTAL _____

### WEIGHT

_____ Binge eating/drinking

_____ Craving certain foods

_____ Excessive weight

_____ Compulsive eating

_____ Water retention

_____ Underweight

TOTAL _____

### OTHER

_____ Frequent illness

_____ Frequent or urgent urination

_____ Genital itch or discharge

TOTAL _____

**GRAND TOTAL** _____

### KEY TO QUESTIONNAIRE

1. Add individual scores and total each group.
2. Add each group score for a grand total.

| | |
|---|---|
| **Optimal** | is less than 10 |
| **Mild toxicity** | 10–50 |
| **Moderate toxicity** | 50–100 |
| **Severe toxicity** | over 100 |

# THE DANIEL PLAN DETOX

Meals that require a recipe are in **bold**; you will find the recipes on pages 304–31.

| | DAY 1 | DAY 2 | DAY 3 | DAY 4 | DAY 5 |
|---|---|---|---|---|---|
| BREAKFAST | **Dr. Hyman's whole food protein shake** | Avocado & veggie 2-egg omelet | 1 cup cooked quinoa with ½ c. unsweetened almond milk and cinnamon | Chia coconut brown rice breakfast bowl | Quinoa breakfast bake |
| SNACK | Mixed veggie sticks (celery, carrots, cucumber, jicama) and ⅓ c. **artichoke hummus** | ½ c. mixed berries plus 25 **cinnamon-toasted almonds** | **Blueberry, spinach, & flax smoothie** | 2 tbsp. **crunchy chickpeas** with hardboiled egg | Veggie mocktail |
| LUNCH | ½ c. quinoa with steamed broccoli and carrots and **antioxidant salad dressing** | 3 turkey roll ups (2 slices low-sodium, nitrate free turkey breast, romaine lettuce, & ⅓ c. **artichoke hummus** | **Dr. Hyman's black bean soup** | **Dr. Hyman's sun-dried tomato turkey burgers** | **Dr. Hyman's raw kale salad** |
| SNACK | Veggie mocktail | 2 tbsp. **crunchy chickpeas** with hardboiled egg | 1 c. steamed organic edamame in the shell | ½ c. mixed berries plus 25 **cinnamon-toasted almonds** | Mixed veggie sticks (celery, carrots, cucumber, jicama) and 2 tbsp. **artichoke hummus** |
| DINNER | Thai-inspired stir fry with coconut rice | **Crockpot beef and veggie stew** | Grilled salmon with cilantro mint chutney with lemon and olive oil quinoa | **Dr. Hyman's walnut pesto chicken** with white beans, chopped peppers, and balsamic vinegar | Shrimp curry with snap peas and water chestnuts |

# THE DANIEL PLAN DETOX cont.

Meals that require a recipe are in **bold**; you will find the recipes on pages 304–31.

| | DAY 6 | DAY 7 | DAY 8 | DAY 9 | DAY 10 |
|---|---|---|---|---|---|
| **BREAKFAST** | 2-egg scramble with spinach, avocado, & tomato | **Dr. Hyman's whole food protein shake** | **Quinoa breakfast bake** | **Blueberry & spinach flax smoothie** | 2 hardboiled eggs with 2 slices nitrate-free turkey and ¼ of avocado |
| **SNACK** | **Blueberry, spinach, flax smoothie** | **Creamy carrot dip** with steamed veggies | 1 c. steamed organic edamame with soy sauce or tamari | **Garlicky white bean dip** with broccoli and carrots | ½ cup mixed berries with 25 **cinnamon-toasted almonds** |
| **LUNCH** | **Dr. Hyman's black bean soup** | **Dr. Hyman's raw kale salad** | 3 turkey roll ups (2 slices low-sodium, nitrate-free turkey breast, romaine lettuce, & ⅓ c. **artichoke hummus**) | **Herbed fish salad** with mixed greens | **Baked broccoli frittata** with mixed greens and **antioxidant salad dressing** |
| **SNACK** | **Garlicky white bean dip** with broccoli and cauliflower | 4 tbsp. crunchy chickpeas | **Dr. Hyman's whole food protein shake** | 2 hardboiled eggs with salt, pepper, chili powder or garlic powder | **Creamy carrot dip** with steamed veggies |
| **DINNER** | **Thai-inspired stir fry** with coconut rice | **Grilled fish with spicy raw slaw** | **Lamb kofta** with cauliflower mash | **Chicken primavera bowl** and steamed green beans | **Greek baked cod** with roasted asparagus and lemon and olive oil quinoa |

# SHOPPING LIST
## for the Daniel Plan Detox

### FRESH PRODUCE

- [ ] 1 banana*
- [ ] 1 large container fresh or frozen blueberries*
- [ ] 4 lemons*
- [ ] 1 lime*
- [ ] 1 bunch asparagus
- [ ] 2 avocados*
- [ ] 1 bunch fresh basil*
- [ ] 2 red bell peppers*
- [ ] 1 small beet
- [ ] 1 head broccoli*
- [ ] 1 head purple or green cabbage†
- [ ] 1 bag carrots*
- [ ] 1 head cauliflower†
- [ ] 1 bag celery
- [ ] 1 bunch cilantro
- [ ] 2 cucumbers
- [ ] 1 bulb garlic*

- [ ] 1 small ginger root
- [ ] 2 cups fresh green beans†
- [ ] 1 jicama
- [ ] 1 package or head of kale
- [ ] 1 bunch fresh mint
- [ ] 1 medium onion
- [ ] 1 red onion*
- [ ] 1 bunch parsley
- [ ] 2 medium purple or sweet potatoes or 1 turnip
- [ ] 1 head romaine lettuce*
- [ ] 2 bags (8–9 oz.) of fresh baby spinach, or one small bunch*
- [ ] 1 pound snap peas
- [ ] 1 cup snow peas or green beans*
- [ ] 1 package grape or cherry tomatoes†
- [ ] 1 zucchini

### MEAT/FISH

- [ ] 1 pound chicken breasts or cutlets*
- [ ] 1 pound lean ground turkey or beef
- [ ] 3–4 pounds chuck roast
- [ ] 1 pound ground lamb†

- [ ] ½ pound sliced turkey breast, nitrate-free*
- [ ] 1 pound hearty white fish†
- [ ] 1 to 1¼ pounds wild salmon
- [ ] 1½ pounds wild shrimp

* Marks items you will use in Days 1–5 and need to repurchase for Days 6–10

† Indicates an ingredient that is required only for Days 6–10

## EGGS

☐ 1 dozen cage-free or organic eggs*

## PASTAS, GRAINS, LEGUMES

☐ 1 package quinoa

☐ 1 package jasmine brown rice or black rice

## FREEZER SECTION

☐ 1 package mixed frozen berries

☐ 1 package frozen organic edamame

## CANS/JARS

☐ 1 can artichokes in water

☐ 2 15-ounce cans low-sodium beef broth

☐ 2 15-ounce cans black beans

☐ 1 15-ounce can white beans†

☐ 2 cans garbanzo beans/chickpeas

☐ 1 jar kalamata or black olives

☐ 1 jar/package sun-dried tomatoes

☐ 1 small can tomato paste

☐ 1 can/box low-sodium vegetable broth

☐ 1 can water chestnuts

## CONDIMENTS/SAUCES

☐ 1 bottle unfiltered apple cider vinegar

☐ 1 bottle balsamic vinegar

☐ 1 container coconut oil or grape seed oil

☐ 1 bottle Dijon mustard

☐ 1 bottle extra-virgin olive oil (or cooking spray)

☐ 1 small bottle rice vinegar

☐ 1 small bottle sesame tahini paste

☐ 1 small bottle gluten-free soy sauce or tamari

* Marks items you will use in Days 1–5 and need to repurchase for Days 6–10
† Indicates an ingredient that is required only for Days 6–10

## NUTS/SEEDS

☐ 1 package ground flax meal/seeds

☐ 1 box unsweetened almond milk

☐ 1 bag raw almonds

☐ 1 jar almond or other nut butter

☐ 1 package chia seeds

☐ 1 small package Brazil nuts

☐ 1 box unsweetened coconut milk*

☐ 1 bag unsweetened shredded coconut

☐ 1 package hemp seeds

☐ 1 small package pine nuts

☐ 1 small package pumpkin seeds

☐ 1 bag raw walnuts

## MISCELLANEOUS

☐ Cornstarch

☐ Currants

☐ 1 container quality protein powder

☐ 1 package organic tempeh*
(usually in the refrigerator section)

## SPICES/HERBS

☐ Bay leaves

☐ Black pepper

☐ Cayenne pepper

☐ Cinnamon

☐ Chili powder

☐ Cumin

☐ Dried oregano

☐ Dry mustard

☐ Garlic powder

☐ Kosher or sea salt

☐ Onion powder

☐ Paprika

☐ Vanilla extract

* Marks items you will use in Days 1–5 and need to repurchase for Days 6–10

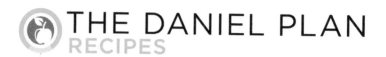

# THE DANIEL PLAN
## RECIPES

**D** INDICATES DETOX-COMPATIBLE RECIPES

## ANTIOXIDANT SALAD DRESSING **D**

¼ cup raw unfiltered apple cider vinegar

2 tablespoons extra-virgin olive, grape seed, or coconut oil

1 clove garlic, crushed

2 tablespoons lemon juice, plus 1 teaspoon grated zest

1 teaspoon ground flax seed

1 teaspoon dry mustard

½ teaspoon oregano

Ground black pepper and salt to taste

**BRISKLY WHISK TOGETHER** vinegar and oil until mixed well (or you can put them in a closed container and shake vigorously). Add remaining ingredients, and whisk (or shake) together until well incorporated. You can vary this dressing to suit your taste by adding other herbs and spices such as basil, tarragon, rosemary, and dill.

*Serves 3 – 4*

## ARTICHOKE HUMMUS **D**

1 (15-ounce) can chickpeas/garbanzo beans

1 cup artichoke hearts, drained and chopped

2 cloves fresh garlic, crushed

2 tablespoons lemon juice

1 tablespoon olive oil

1 tablespoon water

1 tablespoon sesame tahini

Ground black pepper and salt to taste

**COMBINE ALL INGREDIENTS** in a food processor and pulse until smooth. Transfer to a bowl. Chill and serve with mixed veggie sticks such as celery, jicama, and carrots.   *Serves 8 (⅓ cup each)*

## BABA GANOUSH DIP ⓓ

- 1 large eggplant
- ¼ cup tahini, plus more as needed
- 3 garlic cloves, minced
- ¼ cup fresh lemon juice, plus more as needed
- 1 pinch ground cumin
- 1 pinch salt
- 1 tablespoon chopped fresh flat-leaf parsley

**PREHEAT OVEN TO 375°.** Prick the eggplant with a fork in several places and place on a baking sheet. Bake until very soft, about 20 to 30 minutes. Remove from the oven, let cool slightly. Peel off and discard the skin. Place the eggplant flesh in a bowl. Using a fork, mash the eggplant well. Add the tahini, garlic, lemon juice, and cumin, and mix well. Season with salt, then taste and add more tahini and/or lemon juice, if needed. Transfer the mixture to a serving bowl. Sprinkle parsley over the top. Serve at room temperature.   *Serves 4 (¼ cup each)*

## BAKED BROCCOLI FRITTATA

- 6 large eggs
- 1 medium red onion, diced fine
- 1 clove garlic, crushed
- 1 tablespoon fresh parsley, chopped
- 2 cups broccoli, chopped
- Dash of salt
- ¼ teaspoon ground black pepper
- 1 teaspoon extra-virgin olive oil
- 3 tablespoons Parmesan cheese

**PREHEAT OVEN TO 350°.** Heat olive oil in a wide non-stick frying pan over medium heat. Add onion and cook, stirring often, until onion begins to soften (about 3 minutes). Stir in garlic, parsley, and broccoli. Continue cooking, stirring often, until broccoli is bright green (about 3 minutes). Season with salt and pepper. In a large bowl, beat eggs well. Stir in broccoli mixture. Grease shallow 2-quart baking dish. Pour the broccoli mixture into the dish. Sprinkle evenly with Parmesan cheese. Bake uncovered 25 to 30 minutes, until frittata is firm in center when touched.    *Serves 3*

## BERRY PROTEIN SHAKE

    ½ cup mixed frozen berries

    1 cup unsweetened coconut milk

    1 scoop unsweetened protein powder

    1 tablespoon almond butter

    ¼ cup plain Greek yogurt

    ½ cup crushed ice

**COMBINE FIRST FIVE INGREDIENTS** in a blender. Add ice. Blend until smooth.    *Serves 1*

## BLUEBERRY AND SPINACH FLAX SMOOTHIE Ⓓ

    2 cups unsweetened almond or coconut milk

    2 tablespoons ground flax seeds

    1 scoop unsweetened protein powder

    1 cup spinach

    ½ cup fresh or frozen blueberries

    ½ cup crushed ice

**PROCESS FIRST FIVE INGREDIENTS** in a blender. Add ice and process until smooth.    *Serves 2*

## CARROT AND AVOCADO SOUP

   2 teaspoons grape seed oil

   ½ red onion, finely chopped

   2–3 large carrots, steamed and chopped

   1 small avocado, halved and pit removed

   1 teaspoon fresh ginger, minced

   1¾ cup vegetable broth

   14 ounces unsweetened coconut milk

   2 teaspoons cornstarch

   Salt

**IN A MEDIUM SAUCEPAN,** sauté onion until translucent. In a blender, combine onion, carrots, avocado, ginger, broth, and coconut milk. Process until smooth and creamy. Add to saucepan, and mix in cornstarch. Heat for about 5 minutes. Serve at warm or room temperature. *Serves 4*

## CAULIFLOWER MASH Ⓓ

   1 medium cauliflower, trimmed and diced

   2 tablespoons extra-virgin olive oil

   Salt and ground black pepper

**BRING A LARGE POT** of water to a boil. Add cauliflower and cook until very tender, about 10 minutes. Reserve ¼ cup of the cooking liquid and then drain well. In a large bowl, mash cauliflower with reserved water with a potato masher or large fork until smooth but with texture. Add oil, and combine well. Season with salt and pepper. Experiment with herbs and spices in this dish, such as rosemary, thyme, or curry powder. *Serves 6*

## CHIA COCONUT BROWN RICE BREAKFAST Ⓓ

- 1 cup cooked brown rice
- 2 ounces dry chia seeds
- 2 cups coconut milk
- 2 tablespoons coconut flakes

**COMBINE INGREDIENTS** in a container, and refrigerate at least 1 hour. Enjoy warm or cold.

*Serves 3 – 4*

## CHIA COCONUT OATMEAL

- 1 cup steel cut or old-fashioned oats
- 2 ounces dry chia seeds
- 2 cups unsweetened coconut milk
- 1 teaspoon stevia extract
- 2 tablespoons unsweetened coconut flakes

**SOAK OATS AND CHIA SEEDS** in coconut milk overnight. Before eating, warm oatmeal on a stovetop or cook it for about 5 minutes until desired consistency. Stir in stevia, and top it with coconut flakes or shredded coconut. Enjoy warm or cold. Tip: Soaking oatmeal overnight is an easy way to make and enjoy raw or steel cut oatmeal.

*Serves 3*

## CHICKEN PRIMAVERA BOWL Ⓓ

- 4 teaspoons coconut oil
- ¼ large red onion, chopped
- 1 pound chicken breast, boneless, diced into 1-inch pieces
- 1 medium red bell pepper, chopped
- 1 cup grape tomatoes, halved
- 1 cup carrot, grated
- ½ cup parsley, chopped
- 1 teaspoon ground black pepper
- 2 tablespoons lemon juice

IN A LARGE SAUTÉ PAN, cook onions over medium heat in coconut oil until translucent, about 5 minutes. Add chicken and cook until well done, about 8–10 minutes. Add bell pepper, tomatoes, and carrots and cook for another 5 minutes. Top with parsley, ground pepper, and lemon juice and toss again. Serve hot or cold.

VEGGIE COMBO ALTERNATIVES: red kale, zucchini, and cauliflower; broccoli, yellow squash, and fennel; or broiled Japanese eggplant, cauliflower, and snap peas.            *Serves 4*

## CINNAMON TOASTED ALMONDS ⓓ

1 cup raw whole almonds

1 teaspoon ground cinnamon

Extra-virgin olive oil cooking spray

PREHEAT OVEN TO 350°. On a rimmed baking sheet, spread almonds onto a single layer and spray lightly with cooking spray. Sprinkle sifted cinnamon over almonds and bake for about 8–10 minutes or until fragrant. Enjoy warm.            *Serves 4*

## CHOCOLATE AND WALNUT DIPPED FROZEN BANANA POPS

8 ounces of 70% or higher dark chocolate,
   broken into pieces or chunks

2 bananas, cut in half

2 tablespoons crushed walnuts

4 wooden skewers or popsicle sticks

MELT CHOCOLATE in a double boiler or microwave. If using a microwave, be careful not to "cook" the chocolate; nuke it for 30 seconds at a time until soft and gooey. Let chocolate sit for about 5 minutes to cool slightly. Place crushed walnuts on a plate. Thread banana onto skewer or popsicle stick. Dip half of banana into melted chocolate and roll carefully into crushed walnuts. Repeat until all banana pieces are dipped. Place dipped bananas onto a tray lined with wax paper, and freeze for at least 4 hours, preferably overnight.                                    *Serves 4*

## CITRUS MARINADE FOR CHICKEN OR SALMON SKEWERS/VEGGIES

    1 lemon, juiced plus 1 teaspoon zest

    2 limes, juiced plus 1 teaspoon zest

    1 tablespoons balsamic vinegar

    2 teaspoons olive oil

    Ground black pepper and salt

    2 pounds of chicken, salmon, or veggies, cut into 2-inch pieces

**WHISK TOGETHER** first five ingredients until well incorporated. Place chicken, salmon, or veggies separately in marinade. Marinate for at least 1 hour, up to overnight for the chicken or veggies, before cooking. Thread chicken, salmon, and veggies onto skewers and grill or bake until thoroughly cooked. This will make enough for one lunch and one dinner for two people. Make one batch with chicken and one with fish for Days 1–5.     *Serves 4–5*

## CONFETTI SALSA

    2 whole tomatoes, finely diced

    ½ cup frozen corn, thawed

    1 jalapeno pepper, seeded and minced
       (seeds are very spicy; handle with care)

    ½ medium red onion, minced

    3 tablespoons fresh cilantro, minced

    2 limes, juiced, and ¼ teaspoon zest

    Dash of salt

**COMBINE** tomatoes, fresh corn, red onion, jalapeno, cilantro, lime juice, and a dash of salt in a medium bowl. Chill for at least 1 hour.

                                                    *Serves 4*

## CREAMY CARROT DIP ⓓ

1 cup carrots, chopped

2 cloves garlic, crushed

2 lemons, juiced

3 tablespoons extra-virgin olive oil

Dash of salt

¼ teaspoon cayenne pepper

**STEAM CARROTS** until soft, then puree in a food processor. Add other ingredients, puree until smooth, then serve with baked whole grain chips or cut up broccoli and cauliflower. You may adjust the amount of salt and cayenne to taste.   *Serves 4*

## CROCKPOT BEEF AND VEGGIE STEW ⓓ

4 pounds chuck roast, cut into 2-inch cubes

½ cup cornstarch

2 tablespoons grape seed oil

1 large red onion, diced

4 cups low sodium beef broth

1 (6-ounce) can tomato paste

2 cups red-skinned or purple potatoes, chopped
     (turnip or sweet potato can be substituted)

1 cup carrots, chopped

1 cup celery, chopped

1 bay leaf

2 teaspoons ground black pepper

1 teaspoon salt

**ON A PLATE,** spread a thin layer of cornstarch. Roll beef chunks until lightly coated. In a large skillet, heat oil. Brown meat with onions, about 6 – 8 minutes. Add tomato paste and beef broth and combine until well incorporated.

Transfer mixture to crock pot with vegetables and seasonings. Cover and cook over low heat for about 8 hours or on high for 4 hours.   *Serves 4 – 6*

## CRUNCHBERRY YOGURT PARFAIT

  1 pint blueberries

  2 teaspoons pure vanilla extract

  2 tablespoons lemon juice

  1 cup low-sugar granola

  ½ cup walnuts

  32 ounces plain Greek yogurt

  1 teaspoon stevia extract

  4–6 leaves fresh mint

**IN A FOOD PROCESSOR,** puree berries until smooth and transfer to a bowl. Add vanilla extract, lemon juice, and stevia to the berry puree. Chill until ready to assemble parfaits. In individual glasses, layer a few spoonfuls of yogurt, a spoonful of berry mixture, then sprinkle with walnuts. Repeat. Top with fresh mint.    *Serves 4–6*

## CRUNCHY CHICKPEAS Ⓓ

  4 cups garbanzo beans, drained and rinsed

  2 teaspoons extra-virgin olive oil

  1 teaspoon ground cumin

  1 teaspoon ground chili powder

  ½ teaspoon cayenne pepper

**PREHEAT OVEN TO 400°,** and arrange a rack in the middle. Place the chickpeas in a large bowl and toss with the remaining ingredients until evenly coated. Spread the chickpeas in an even layer on a rimmed baking sheet and bake until crisp, about 30 to 40 minutes.    *Serves 12 (1 ounce each)*

## CRUNCHY MEDITERRANEAN SALAD WITH GRILLED SHRIMP

  1 pound wild caught shrimp, peeled and deveined

  1 tablespoon grape seed oil

  2 cups romaine lettuce, shredded

2 cups baby spinach

1 medium tomato, chopped

½ cucumber, chopped

4 tablespoons fresh parsley, chopped

⅛ large red onion, sliced thinly

2 tablespoons feta cheese

8 kalamata or black olives

2 tablespoons **antioxidant salad dressing** (see recipe, p. 304)

⅓ cup **crunchy chickpeas** (see recipe, p. 312)

**BRUSH SHRIMP** with grape seed oil. Grill in a hot grill pan for about 2 minutes on each side or until bright pink. Chop lettuce, spinach, and parsley into bite-size pieces. Chop tomato and cucumber. Combine all vegetable ingredients in a bowl. Toss with 2 tablespoons of the salad dressing. Top with grilled shrimp and crunchy chickpeas. *Serves 2*

## DARK CHOCOLATE AVOCADO MOUSSE CUP

⅔ cup of 70% or higher dark chocolate, chopped

1 tablespoon coconut oil

1 teaspoon stevia extract

1 tablespoon brewed coffee

½ teaspoon pure vanilla extract

1 avocado

**TOPPING:** ½ cup whole strawberries or toasted almonds (optional)

**MELT CHOCOLATE** in a double boiler or microwave. If using a microwave, be careful not to "cook" the chocolate; nuke it at 30 seconds at a time until soft and gooey. Add coconut oil, sweetener, coffee, and vanilla extract to melted chocolate, and mix well. Scoop out avocado and blend it into the chocolate mixture. You can use a hand or stick blender to achieve a smooth consistency. Scoop out into 4 equal portions and chill for at least 2 hours. Top with a spoon of toasted almonds or strawberries before serving. *Serves 4*

## DARK CHOCOLATE TRAIL MIX

½ cup raw unsalted almonds

½ cup raw unsalted walnuts

½ cup unsalted sunflower seeds

2 ounces dark chocolate chips (70% cocoa or more)

1 cup raisins

1 cup dried blueberries

**COMBINE ALL INGREDIENTS.** Store in an airtight container or bag. *Serves 7 (2 ounces each)*

## DR. HYMAN'S BLACK BEAN SOUP Ⓓ

1 tablespoon extra-virgin olive oil

1 tablespoon garlic

1 small onion, diced

1 tablespoon cumin

2 (15-ounce) cans black beans

2 cups water or vegetable stock

1 bay leaf

1½ tablespoons wheat-free tamari

1 tablespoon lemon juice

Chopped fresh cilantro for garnish

**HEAT THE OLIVE OIL** over medium heat in a soup pot. Add the garlic and onions, and cook until the onions are translucent. Add the cumin, and sauté a few more minutes. Add the canned beans, including their liquid, water or stock, and bay leaf. Bring to a boil, reduce heat, and simmer for 10 – 15 minutes. Add the tamari and lemon juice and simmer 1 minute more. *Serves 5 – 7*

Source: *The Blood Sugar Solution* by Dr. Mark Hyman[1]

## DR. HYMAN'S GRILLED SALMON WITH CILANTRO MINT CHUTNEY Ⓓ

1½ pounds wild salmon

1 tablespoon extra-virgin olive oil

Pinch of salt

Pinch of black pepper

**CHUTNEY:**

1 small bunch cilantro, including stems, rinsed

2 tablespoons fresh mint leaves, chopped

3 tablespoons extra-virgin olive oil

1½ tablespoons garlic, minced

Pinch of salt

1 tablespoon fresh lemon or lime juice

Pinch of chili pepper flakes (optional)

**SEASON THE SALMON** with the olive oil, salt, and pepper. Set aside for 10 minutes. Combine all the chutney ingredients in a blender. Blend until smooth and fragrant. Set aside. Heat a griddle, grill, or grill pan on medium-high heat. Place the fish on the grill, skin side down. Allow the salmon to cook until the skin is charred and the fish is almost cooked through. This will take about 15 minutes, depending on the thickness of the salmon. Turn the salmon over and grill a few more minutes, until the fish is fully cooked. Remove from heat, and lay skin side up on a platter. Pull the skin off the salmon, and flip back to serve. Spread chutney on top of the salmon. Serve with wedges of lemon or lime.   *Serves 4*

Source: *The Blood Sugar Solution* by Dr. Mark Hyman

## DR. HYMAN'S RAW KALE SALAD Ⓓ

1 large bunch kale, stemmed and finely chopped

Zest and juice of 1 large lemon

¼ cup extra-virgin olive oil

1 garlic clove, minced

⅛ teaspoon salt

¼ cup toasted pine nuts

¼ cup currants

½ cup chopped pitted kalamata olives

**PLACE THE KALE** in a large salad bowl, and add the lemon zest and juice, olive oil, garlic, and salt. Massage the mixture with your hands for 1–2 minutes to soften the kale. Add the remaining ingredients and toss to combine. Allow the salad to rest and soften for about 15 minutes before serving. Kale salad is best if eaten the same day, but can be stored overnight in the refrigerator. *Serves 4*

Source: *The Blood Sugar Solution Cookbook* by Dr. Mark Hyman[2]

## DR. HYMAN'S SUN-DRIED TOMATO TURKEY BURGERS Ⓓ

3 tablespoons sun-dried tomatoes

1 teaspoon extra-virgin olive oil

1 pound organic ground turkey meat

1 tablespoon balsamic vinegar

2–3 tablespoons fresh basil, chopped

1 tablespoon garlic, minced

1½ teaspoons Dijon mustard

Pinch of salt

Pinch of black pepper

**COVER THE SUN-DRIED TOMATOES** in warm water and soak until soft. This will take about 10 minutes, depending on how soft your tomatoes are to start with. Drain and chop tomatoes into small pieces. Combine with the remaining ingredients and form into 4 patties. Grill, pan-sear, or bake in the oven at 375° until done, about 8 minutes. Serve over a large salad.  *Serves 4*

Source: *The Blood Sugar Solution* by Dr. Mark Hyman

## DR. HYMAN'S WALNUT PESTO CHICKEN ⓓ

1 pound skinless boneless chicken

Pinch of salt

1 tablespoon grape seed or extra-virgin olive oil

2 tablespoons extra-virgin olive oil

¼ cup raw walnuts

2 cups fresh basil leaves

2 garlic cloves

Pinch of salt (additional)

**SLICE THE CHICKEN** into thin strips. Toss with salt. Heat 1 table-spoon of grape seed or olive oil in sauté pan or griddle over medium-high heat. Cook the chicken on each side until cooked through. Set aside on a paper towel to cool. Grind the walnuts in a food processor until fine. Rinse basil leaves and pat dry. Add the basil, garlic, and salt to the processor. With the processor running, drizzle in 2 tablespoons of olive oil until desired consistency is reached. Toss with the chicken strips. (Unused pesto can be kept in the fridge for up to a week.) Serve with veggies, brown rice, or quinoa, or use as a spread.                                   *Serves 4*

Source: *The Blood Sugar Solution* by Dr. Mark Hyman

## DR. HYMAN'S WHOLE FOOD PROTEIN SHAKE ⓓ

1 cup frozen blueberries

2 tablespoons almond butter

2 tablespoons pumpkin seeds

2 tablespoons chia seeds

2 tablespoons hemp seeds

4 walnuts

3 Brazil nuts

1 large banana

1 tablespoon extra-virgin coconut oil

½ cup unsweetened almond milk

1 cup water

COMBINE ALL OF THE INGREDIENTS in a blender. Blend on high speed until smooth, about 2 minutes. If the shake is too thick, add more water until you reach a thick but drinkable consistency. Serve chilled.                                                                          *Serves 3*

Source: *The Blood Sugar Solution* by Dr. Mark Hyman

## FISH TACOS WITH FRESH PINEAPPLE SALSA

### PINEAPPLE SALSA:

1 cup fresh pineapple, diced (if fresh is unavailable, use canned pineapple and drain juice)

3 tablespoons fresh cilantro, chopped

¼ large red onion, diced fine

½ teaspoon black pepper

1 fresh lime

COMBINE SALSA INGREDIENTS in a bowl, and refrigerate at least 1 hour.

### FISH TACOS:

¾ pound wild-caught halibut or hearty white fish

1 teaspoon extra-virgin olive oil

6 organic corn tortillas

1 cup purple or green cabbage, shredded

1 cup white or black beans (rinse beans before using)

3 tablespoons plain Greek yogurt or sour cream

1 fresh lime, wedged into 6 pieces

BRUSH HALIBUT WITH OLIVE OIL and grill on a hot grill or grill pan until well-cooked, about 8 minutes on each side. Warm corn tortillas for 5–10 minutes in an oven preheated at 350° or on a skillet over medium heat until tortilla is pliable. Layer grilled halibut, beans, pineapple salsa, and cabbage over warm tortilla. Top taco with a tablespoon of sour cream or Greek yogurt, and serve with a wedge of fresh lime to squeeze over top.

*Serves 3 (2 tacos each)*

## FROZEN COCONUT BERRY DESSERT

1 cup mixed frozen berries

1 cup unsweetened coconut milk

1 scoop vanilla protein powder

1 tablespoon ground flax seeds

**COMBINE ALL INGREDIENTS** in a blender. Transfer to a freezer-proof container, and freeze. Scoop and enjoy as a frozen dessert.

*Serves 2*

## GARLICKY WHITE BEAN DIP ⓓ

1 (15-ounce) can cannellini or great northern white beans, rinsed and drained

1 tablespoon extra-virgin olive oil

2 tablespoons water

4 small garlic cloves, crushed

Juice of 1 lemon

1 teaspoon paprika

**IN A FOOD PROCESSOR,** pulse beans with olive oil and water until smooth. Add crushed garlic, lemon juice, and paprika and pulse until creamy texture is achieved. Serve with your favorite raw vegetables.

*Serves 6 (2 ounces each)*

## GLUTEN-FREE TORTILLA CHIPS

6 organic corn tortillas

Olive oil cooking spray

Salt

2 teaspoons ground cumin

**PREHEAT OVEN TO 375°.** Cut corn tortillas in six triangles. Spray cooking spray onto a baking sheet. Arrange tortilla chips on baking sheet in a single layer. Spray chips with olive oil. Bake for 15 minutes or until tortillas are golden and crisp. Sprinkle cumin on chips.

*Serves 3*

## GRAPEFRUIT AND POMEGRANATE SEED SALAD WITH COCONUT

    1 medium pink grapefruit
    ½ cup pomegranate seeds
    Juice of 1 orange
    1 tablespoon shredded unsweetened coconut

**PEEL GRAPEFRUIT** and cut it into bite sizes. Remove pomegranate seeds from pomegranate. (You can also buy pomegranate seeds ready to use.) In a mixing bowl combine grapefruit, pomegranate, and coconut. Add the juice of one orange. Mix well. Serve cold.                                    *Serves 2*


## GREEK BAKED COD ⓓ

    1 pound cod or firm white fish
    2 cloves garlic, crushed
    ½ cup red onion, finely chopped
    10 kalamata olives, pitted
    1 teaspoon extra-virgin olive oil
    1 teaspoon salt
    1 teaspoon ground black pepper
    1 tablespoon fresh oregano (or 1 teaspoon dried)
    Juice of 1 lemon

**CHOP ONION, GARLIC, OREGANO, AND OLIVES.** In a small bowl, add olive oil, lemon juice, salt, and pepper to chopped veggies. You can use a food processor to chop and combine all marinated ingredients. In a large bowl or large plastic bag, add fish and marinate for 30 minutes to 1 hour. When time to cook, preheat the oven to 350°. Place the fish in a greased ovenproof pan/dish. Bake for 20 to 30 minutes until the fish flakes easily.    *Serves 3*

## GREEK YOGURT WITH NO-SUGAR-ADDED MUESLI

### YOGURT

6 ounces Greek yogurt

1 teaspoon raw honey

### MUESLI

2 tablespoons rolled oats

1 teaspoon raisins

2 tablespoons dried blueberries

1 tablespoon slivered almonds

**COMBINE ALL MUESLI INGREDIENTS.** In a dessert glass, layer yogurt, raw honey, then muesli mix.                    *Serves 1*

## GRILLED FISH WITH SPICY RAW SLAW Ⓓ

1 pound wild caught halibut or hearty white fish

1 teaspoon extra-virgin olive oil

Dash of salt and ground pepper

2 cups purple or green cabbage, shredded

1 cup carrots, shredded

2 tablespoons organic smooth almond or other nut butter

2 teaspoons rice wine vinegar

½ teaspoon cayenne pepper

Juice of 1 lime

**BRUSH HALIBUT WITH OLIVE OIL,** sprinkle with salt and pepper. Grill on a hot grill or grill pan until flaky, about 8 minutes on each side. In a separate bowl, combine nut butter, rice wine vinegar, cayenne, and lime juice. Toss with cabbage and carrots. Serve fish on top of spicy slaw.                    *Serves 3*

## GRILLED MEDITERRANEAN LAMB KOFTA ⓓ

    3 cloves garlic, crushed

    2 tablespoons onion, grated

    ¼ cup fresh parsley, chopped

    1 teaspoon salt

    2 teaspoons ground black pepper

    1 teaspoon allspice

    1 teaspoon paprika

    1 tablespoon ground coriander

    1 pound ground lamb

    Wooden or metal skewers

**PREHEAT GRILL TO MEDIUM HEAT.** (You can also forgo the skewers and shape lamb into sausages and cook over medium heat in a sauté pan.) In a large bowl, combine crushed garlic, spices, and seasonings and, working with hands, incorporate into ground lamb until well blended.

Form seasoned lamb mixture into a sausage-like shape around skewers. If using wooden skewers, make sure to soak the skewers in water for at least 30 minutes before placing on grill. Cook kofta skewers on the preheated grill, turning occasionally, for about 7 – 8 minutes or until desired doneness.                 *Serves 3 – 4*

## GROUND TURKEY AND BROCCOLI PASTA

    ¾ pound ground turkey

    2 cups gluten-free pasta

    1 head of broccoli

    ½ cup chopped onion

    2 medium tomatoes, diced

    1 teaspoon yellow mustard

    1 tablespoon low-sodium soy sauce

    1 teaspoon salt

    1 teaspoon ground black pepper

    1 teaspoon extra-virgin olive oil

IN A LARGE SAUCEPAN, bring 8–10 cups of water to a boil. Add pasta and cook for 10 minutes or just until pasta is cooked through.

Preheat a large skillet. Drizzle olive oil. Add ground turkey, and cook until golden brown.

Add chopped onions to turkey. Cook for 5 minutes until onions are translucent. Add chopped tomatoes, broccoli, mustard, soy sauce, salt, and pepper. Cook until broccoli is tender, but not mushy, and the ingredients have created a light sauce on the bottom of pan.

In a large bowl, combine pasta with turkey sauce. Serve at warm or room temperature.                                    *Serves 3*

## GROUND TURKEY STUFFED BELL PEPPERS  Ⓓ

3 large red bell peppers

¾ pound lean ground turkey

½ cup chopped onions

½ cup chopped parsley

2 tomatoes, diced

1 teaspoon extra-virgin olive oil

Pinch of salt

1 teaspoon ground black pepper

PREHEAT THE OVEN TO 375°. Cut bell peppers in half lengthwise. Chop onion, tomatoes, and parsley. Heat olive oil in a nonstick skillet over medium high heat. Add turkey and cook until golden brown.

Add onions, salt, and pepper to turkey. Cook until onion is translucent. Add diced tomatoes. Cook until tomatoes are soft and incorporated into dish. Add parsley. Stuff bell pepper halves with turkey mixture. Place stuffed peppers in a shallow nonstick pan lined with foil. Cook for 30 minutes until pepper is tender.

*Serves 3*

## HERBED FISH SALAD Ⓓ

8 ounces canned/packaged fish, such as salmon or
low-mercury tuna

2 tablespoons fresh dill

Juice of 1 lemon

1 teaspoon garlic powder

1 tablespoon organic or vegan mayonnaise

Pinch of salt and pepper

2 celery stalks, finely diced

**COMBINE INGREDIENTS IN A BOWL,** and serve chilled. *Serves 2*

## LIGHT PUMPKIN PIE SQUARES

### CRUST

1½ cups almond meal/flour

3 tablespoons coconut oil (room temperature)

1 tablespoon cinnamon

½ cup rolled oats

**HEAT OVEN TO 350°.** In a medium bowl, mix ingredients until a well-combined consistency is created. Grease a 9-by-9 nonstick pan. Press crust mixture into pan. Bake for 10 – 12 minutes or until the crust becomes light brown. Remove from oven.

### FILLING

18 ounces extra-firm organic tofu

2 cups canned (or cooked) pumpkin

1 cup Greek yogurt

2 teaspoons stevia extract

1 teaspoon pure vanilla extract

2 teaspoons pumpkin pie spice

**PREHEAT OVEN TO 350°.** Drain tofu. Place in a food processor, and process until smooth. Add remaining filling ingredients. Process until well blended. Pour onto crust, and bake for about an hour or until a toothpick comes out clean. Remove from oven and cool completely. Then chill until firm. Cut into squares and dust with cinnamon.

*Serves 9*

## MANGO COCONUT POWER SMOOTHIE

- 1 cup frozen or fresh mango
- 1 cup unsweetened coconut milk
- 1 cup water
- 1 scoop protein powder, unsweetened
- 1 scoop ice

**COMBINE INGREDIENTS IN A BLENDER.** Add ice and blend until smooth. Serve cold.

*Serves 1*

## NO-BAKE POWER BITES

- 1 cup rolled oats
- ½ cup unsweetened shredded coconut plus ⅓ cup for topping
- 1 scoop chocolate protein powder
- 2 tablespoons natural almond or other nut butter
- ½ cup ground flax meal
- ½ cup dark chocolate chips (70% or more cocoa powder)
- 1 teaspoon stevia extract
- ⅔ cup unsweetened coconut milk
- 1 teaspoon pure vanilla extract

**IN A SMALL BOWL,** mix all ingredients thoroughly. Chill in the refrigerator for an hour. Roll into 2-inch balls, then roll in shredded coconut. Set balls on wax paper in an airtight container in the refrigerator or freezer.

Allow to rest at room temperature for 5 minutes before eating.

*Serves 20 – 25 (1 ball each)*

## QUINOA BREAKFAST BAKE ⓓ

   1½ cups red or white quinoa, rinsed

   2 eggs

   ⅓ cup unsweetened coconut or almond milk

   1 teaspoon vanilla extract

   1 tablespoon cinnamon

   2 tablespoons almond butter

   1 teaspoon stevia extract

**TO COOK QUINOA:** Bring 3 cups of water to a boil. Add ½ teaspoon of salt and 1½ cups of quinoa. Simmer for about 20 minutes, or until quinoa is cooked and water is completely absorbed. Cool quinoa. Preheat the oven to 375°, and place the quinoa in a large mixing bowl. Grease an 8-by-8-inch baking pan. In a small bowl, whisk together eggs, coconut milk, vanilla extract, and cinnamon until thoroughly combined. Add stevia and whisk. Add egg mixture to cooked and cooled quinoa. Stir with a large spoon to combine. Pour into the baking dish and spread it around to ensure that it's even. Bake for 20 to 25 minutes until set and golden. Cool completely and cut into squares. Serve with a dollop of nut butter.

*Serves 6*

## SAVORY OVEN-FRIED CHICKEN

   12 natural chicken legs

   2 cups buttermilk (omit for detox recipe)

   1 tablespoon Dijon mustard
      (increase to 6 tablespoons for detox recipe)

   1½ cups ground flax seeds

   1 teaspoon cayenne pepper

   1 teaspoon dried oregano

   1 tablespoon onion powder

   1 tablespoon garlic powder

   2 tablespoons ground black pepper

   Salt

IN A MEDIUM BOWL, mix buttermilk and mustard, immerse chicken pieces in buttermilk, and soak for at least 30 minutes or up to 8 hours. Combine flax meal with herbs and spices on a flat plate. Remove chicken pieces from buttermilk, and shake off excess liquid. Roll chicken pieces in flax meal crumb mixture until thoroughly coated. Place chicken in a lightly sprayed baking pan or on a baking sheet. Bake at 400° for about 40 minutes, covered with foil to keep moist. Remove cover for final 10 – 15 minutes until crust is golden brown. Internal temperature of chicken should be at least 165°.

DETOX ALTERNATIVE: Omit buttermilk; instead, brush chicken with Dijon mustard, then roll in the flax meal crumb mixture.

*Serves 6*

## SHRIMP CURRY WITH SNAP PEAS AND WATER CHESTNUTS Ⓓ

2 tablespoons coconut oil

2 tablespoons curry powder

2 pounds wild caught shrimp, peeled and deveined

1 pound sugar snap peas, trimmed

½ cup water chestnuts

1 cup unsweetened coconut milk

Juice of 2 limes

Dash of sea salt

2 teaspoons cornstarch

IN A LARGE SKILLET OR WOK, heat coconut oil over medium heat. Add curry powder and cook until fragrant, about 1 minute. Add shrimp and sugar snap peas, and cook about 2 minutes. Add water chestnuts, coconut milk, lime juice, and salt. Whisk cornstarch in until fully dissolved and sauce thickens slightly, about 5 minutes. Serve with cooked brown rice or quinoa.   *Serves 4*

## STRAWBERRY COCO CHOCO SHAKE

1 cup frozen strawberries

1 cup unsweetened coconut milk

1 scoop chocolate protein powder

1 tablespoon ground flax seed

1 scoop ice

**COMBINE INGREDIENTS IN A BLENDER.** Add ice and blend until smooth. Serve cold.                                                   *Serves 1*

## SUPERCHARGED BULGUR WHEAT BREAKFAST BOWL

1 cup whole grain bulgur wheat

2 cups water

1 cup unsweetened coconut milk

½ cup unsweetened applesauce

½ cup unsweetened coconut flakes

½ cup slivered almonds

**BRING WATER TO A BOIL.** Add bulgur wheat, and simmer for about 20 minutes. Transfer to a medium bowl. Add coconut milk and applesauce. Mix with a spoon. Top with coconut and almonds. Serve hot or at room temperature for breakfast or chilled in a champagne glass.                                                   *Serves 4*

## SUPER GREENS WATERMELON SALAD

2 cups arugula

2 cups kale, chopped

2 cups spinach

1 cup watermelon, diced (or grapefruit)

1 tablespoon toasted unsalted sunflower seeds

**Antioxidant salad dressing** (see recipe, p. 304)

**CHOP KALE TO BITE-SIZE PIECES.** (Tip: Stack kale leaves into a pile. Roll the leaves together. Run a sharp knife through roll of kale to create thin to medium strips). Chop watermelon into cubes. Mix arugula, spinach, and kale together. Add watermelon cubes to salad. Drizzle with 2 tablespoons of homemade salad dressing. Top with toasted sunflower seeds.                    *Serves 2*

## THAI-INSPIRED STIR FRY WITH COCONUT RICE Ⓓ

### STIR FRY

12 ounces organic tempeh

1 small onion, chopped

3 cloves garlic, crushed

1 cup carrots, diced

1 cup red pepper, diced

1 cup snow peas, diced

1 cup zucchini, diced

1 teaspoon extra-virgin olive oil

2 tablespoons low sodium soy sauce

1 teaspoon black pepper

### RICE

1 cup brown jasmine rice or black rice

1 cup unsweetened coconut milk

1 cup water

**DICE ALL VEGETABLES INTO BITE-SIZE PIECES.** Cut tempeh into 1-inch-long rectangles. Heat olive oil in a skillet over medium heat. Add tempeh, and cook until golden brown. Add vegetables and soy sauce. Stir fry until vegetables are tender, about 5 minutes. To cook rice, bring coconut milk and water to a boil in a medium saucepan. Add rice and reduce heat to low. Cook until all liquid is absorbed, about 25 minutes.                    *Serves 3*

## VEGGIE, LENTIL, AND CHICKEN SAUSAGE SOUP Ⓓ

1 pound lentils, raw

4 links chicken sausage

1 tablespoon olive oil

1 cup onion, chopped

½ cup carrot, chopped

½ cup celery, chopped

1 teaspoon salt

1 teaspoon ground black pepper

¼ teaspoon cayenne pepper

½ teaspoon ground cumin

1 cup canned tomatoes, no salt added

2 quarts organic low-sodium chicken broth

**HEAT OLIVE OIL IN A LARGE SOUP POT** over medium heat. Add onion, carrot, celery, and salt and sweat until the onions are translucent, approximately 5 minutes. Add the lentils, tomatoes, broth, peppers, and cumin. Stir to combine. Increase the heat to high and bring just to a boil. Reduce the heat to low, cover and cook at a low simmer until the lentils are tender, approximately 35 to 40 minutes. Using a sharp knife make a cut on one end of the sausage links. Remove sausage meat from link casing by squeezing meat through the cut on the link. Heat olive oil in a large pan over medium heat. Add sausage meat and cook until golden brown, breaking up the meat as you cook it. Drain any excess fat. Add to finished lentil soup and serve hot.    *Serves 6*

## VEGGIE MOCKTAIL Ⓓ

2 cup fresh spinach

½ small uncooked beet

5 celery stalks, ends trimmed

½ lemon, peeled

½- to 1-inch piece ginger root, peeled

2 cloves fresh garlic

**IN A JUICER,** push through spinach, beet, celery, lemon, ginger, and garlic. Stir the juice and pour into a glass. Serve at room temperature or chilled, as desired.

*Serves 1*

## WHOLE GRAIN SPAGHETTI ALLA LUCCA

  1 tablespoon grape seed oil

  ½ cup chopped onion

  3 garlic cloves, crushed

  1 pound lean chicken sausage, casings removed

  2½ cups tomato puree

  1 red bell pepper, chopped

  4 leaves fresh basil, chopped

  Sea salt and freshly ground black pepper to taste

  1 can cannellini or white beans, drained and rinsed

  ½ cup grated Parmesan cheese (omit for vegan option)

  1 pound whole grain spaghetti (or gluten-free pasta, quinoa, or
    brown rice)

**COAT A LARGE SKILLET** with oil and place over medium-low heat. Add the onion and crushed garlic, cook and stir until translucent, about 5 minutes. Add the sausage. Cook and stir for 5 to 10 minutes until the meat is no longer pink. Place a separate pot over medium-low heat; add the tomato puree, bell pepper, basil, and black pepper. Season with a dash of sea salt. Add the beans. Cover and gently simmer for about 15 minutes. In a large pot, bring salted water to a boil. Add the pasta, give it a stir, and cook until al dente (firm, not mushy). Drain and set aside. In a large bowl, combine the meat mixture and tomato puree mixture. Toss with pasta until uniform. Top with freshly grated Parmesan and serve.

*Serves 4*

# Metric Conversion Chart

The following measurements are approximate metric weight and volume equivalents for common measurements provided in this book. If converting to metric, use the volume amount when the U.S. measurement is given by volume (teaspoon, tablespoon, cup) and use the weight equivalent when the U.S. measurement is given by weight (ounce, pound).

| U.S. MEASUREMENT | METRIC EQUIVALENT |
| --- | --- |
| ¼ cup | 60 milliliters |
| ⅓ cup | 80 milliliters |
| ½ cup | 120 milliliters |
| 1 cup | 8 fluid ounces or 236 milliliters |
| 2 cups | 460 milliliters |
| 1 tablespoon | .5 fluid ounce or 14.8 milliliters |
| 1 teaspoon | 4.9 milliliters |
| 1 ounce | 28.35 grams |
| 1 pound | 453.59 grams |
| ¼ inch | .6 centimeters |
| 1 inch | 2.5 centimeters |

For metric equivalents, use the following general formulas:

- Ounces to grams — multiply ounces by 28.35
- Pounds to grams — multiply pounds by 453.5
- Pounds to kilograms — multiply pounds by .45
- Cups to liters — multiply cups by .24
- Fahrenheit to centigrade — subtract 32 from Fahrenheit temperature, multiply by 5, then divide by 9

# Acknowledgments

With tremendous gratitude, we thank our pastor, Rick Warren, for his heart and vision that ultimately launched The Daniel Plan in January 2011. Rick's love for God and for people combined to start a worldwide movement to help people begin their journey to health and fully live out God's plan and purpose for their lives.

Our founding doctors, Dr. Mark Hyman, Dr. Daniel Amen, and Dr. Mehmet Oz, pioneered The Daniel Plan and made profound contributions that have transformed thousands of lives. Their ongoing support, friendship, medical insight, and passion to help people get well have been priceless gifts to our ministry.

From the beginning, Kathrine Lee greatly contributed to The Daniel Plan as an advisor and organizational strategist. Her love for helping people reach their God-given potential, along with her life coaching skills, have been invaluable. Tana Amen has generously offered her leadership, expertise, and passion to develop key resources for the program. Her nutrition and wellness input helped to set the stage for our current plan.

Karen Quinn is a treasured ambassador for our team, with a "can-do" attitude that is unmatched. She initiated and fostered key strategic relationships and alliances, representing The Daniel Plan in several national forums.

Our three Daniel Plan Signature Chefs — Sally Cameron, Jenny Ross, and Robert Sturm — have infused endless creativity into our Food Essential in offering their time and talents to create numerous recipes, lead hands-on workshops, and inspire people to get back into the kitchen and cook real food. A special thanks to Chef Mareya Ibrahim for her significant contribution in helping to create The Daniel Plan Core and Detox plans.

Our Daniel Plan Fitness Experts — Sean Foy, Jimmy Peña, and Tom Wilson — have helped people discover movement they enjoy to get back into shape. Their passion to combine faith and fitness into our program has helped our community learn how to worship as they get stronger for the glory of God. We are especially thankful to Sean for creating our 40-Day Fitness Plan as well.

To our entire Saddleback Fitness Team: We are grateful for your commitment to the health of our community. Thank you to our instructors who consistently volunteer their time each week — Jim, Tony, Kimberly, Juilianne, Kinzie, Tasha, Janet, Paul, Lisa, Elizabeth, Jennifer — and to their fearless leader, Tracy Jones, who compassionately leads and coordinates the entire team.

Brian Williams has blessed us with developing key life coaching principles for our focus groups and curriculum. We are most grateful to the team of volunteer coaches who made such a significant contribution: Katherine, James, Dr. German, Georgina, April, Mareya, Renata, Darci, Joel, Carmen, Bec, Kalei, Ann, and Kenna.

To our broad community of those many, many volunteers — too numerous to mention by name — who have selflessly given their hearts and gifts to The Daniel Plan, we are thankful for each of you: the workshop team led by Joann, the communication team led by Patti and Lori, the social media team with Tabitha and Jenny, and the Sports/Adventure team led by Ron and Tracy.

The Daniel Plan has benefited from Shelly Antol's unwavering dedication as she oversees operational support and strategic projects. Her decisive, uplifting, and God-centered approach is a pure gift. Our resident writer, April O'Neil, publishes our weekly blog and oversees our website and social media venues. Her desire to help people heal and her servant leadership breathe grace into the overall communications strategy for The Daniel Plan. Kelly Ruiten, our coordinator extraordinaire, puts her loving spirit into everything and everyone she touches.

Her nutrition and wellness input helped to set the stage for our current plan.

Karen Quinn is a treasured ambassador for our team, with a "can do" attitude that is unmatched. She initiated and fostered key strategic relationships and alliances, representing The Daniel Plan in several national forums.

Brian Williams has blessed us with developing key life coaching principles for our focus groups and curriculum. We are most grateful to the team of volunteer coaches who made such a significant contribution: Katherine, James, Dr. German, Georgina, April, Mareya, Renata, Darci, Joel, Carmen, Bec, Kalei, Ann, and Kenna.

To our broad community of those many, many volunteers — too numerous to mention by name — who have selflessly given their heart and gifts to The Daniel Plan, we are thankful for each of you: the workshop team led by Joann, the communication team led by Patti and Lori, the social media team with Tabitha and Jenny, and the Sports/Adventure team led by Ron and Tracy.

Our faith foundation has been infused with support from our pastoral team. We express our heartfelt gratitude to Buddy Owens, Steve Gladen, Tom Holladay, John Baker, David Chrzan, Todd Oltoff, Cody Moran, Dave Barr, and Steve Willis. Your faithful leadership is most appreciated.

# Notes

## CHAPTER 1: HOW IT ALL BEGAN

1. Stephen Adams, "Obesity Killing Three Times as Many as Malnutrition," *The Telegraph*, 13 December 2012. http://www.telegraph.co.uk/health/healthnews/9742960/Obesity-killing-three-times-as-many-as-malnutrition.html

2. Cheryl D. Fryar, et al., *NCHS Health E-Stat: Prevalence of Overweight, Obesity, and Extreme Obesity Among Adults*, Centers for Disease Control and Prevention, 13 September 2012. http://www.cdc.gov/nchs/data/hestat/obesity_adult_09_10/obesity_adult_09_10.htm

3. "UN: Chronic Ailments More Deadly Than Infectious Diseases," CNNhealth.com, 22 May 2008. http://www.cnn.com/2008/HEALTH/05/22/world.death/

4. Howard Robinson, "Dualism," *Stanford Encyclopedia of Philosophy*, 2011. http://plato.stanford.edu/entries/dualism/

## CHAPTER 2: THE ESSENTIALS

1. "Chronic Diseases and Health Promotion," Centers for Disease Control and Prevention, 13 August 2012. http://www.cdc.gov/chronicdisease/overview/index.htm

2. "Chronic Diseases: The Power to Prevent, The Call to Control," Centers for Disease Control and Prevention, 2009. http://www.cdc.gov/chronicdisease/resources/publications/aag/chronic.htm

3. HBO Documentary Films, *The Weight of the Nation*, 2012. https://theweightofthenation.hbo.com/films/bonus-shorts/obesity-research-and-the-national-institutes-of-health

4. "Food Consumption in America: What Are We Eating?" Visual Economics: The Credit Blog, 2010. http://www.creditloan.com/blog/food-consumption-in-america/

5. Martin E. Seligman, *Authentic Happiness* (New York: The Free Press, 2002).

6. "The Two-Month Curse: Don't Let January Workout Resolutions Fade," Inside IU Bloomington, 7 February 2013. http://inside.iub.edu/editors-picks/health -wellness/2013 – 02 – 07-iniub-health-workout.shtml

Laine Williams, "Fitness for Life," Time Inc., 2006. http://www.timeinc.net/ web/partners/pb/fitness_for_life.html

## CHAPTER 3: FAITH

1. Rick Warren, *The Purpose Driven Life: What on Earth Am I Here For?* (Grand Rapids: Zondervan, 2002), 174.

2. "μετάνοια, ας, ή (metanoia)," *Strong's Concordance,* 3341. http://biblesuite.com/ greek/3341.htm

3. Viktor E. Frankl, *Man's Search for Meaning* (Boston: Beacon Press, 1992), 75.

## CHAPTER 4: FOOD

1. Environmental Working Group, "Good Food on a Tight Budget," 12 August 2012. http://www.ewg.org/release/good-food-tight-budget-ewg-s-new-easy -use-guide

2. Ramon Estruch, M.D., Ph.D., et al., "Primary Prevention of Cardiovascular Disease with a Mediterranean Diet," *New England Journal of Medicine,* 25 February 2013. http://www.nejm.org/doi/full/10.1056/NEJMoa12003 03#t=article

3. Magalie Lenoir, Fuschia Serr, et al., "Intense Sweetness Surpasses Cocaine Reward," PLoS ONE, 1 August 2007. http://www.plosone.org/article/fetch Article.action?articleURI=info%3Adoi%2F10.1371%2Fjournal.pone.0000698

4. S. M. Schmid, et al., "A Single Night of Sleep Deprivation Increases Ghrelin Levels and Feelings of Hunger in Normal-Weight Healthy Men," University of Luebeck, PubMed.gov, 17 September 2008. http://www.ncbi.nlm.nih.gov/ pubmed/18564298

5. *The Prince's Speech: On the Future of Food* (New York: Rodale, 2012).

6. American Heart Association, "By Any Other Name It's Still Sweetener." http:// www.heart.org/HEARTORG/Conditions/More/MyHeartandStrokeNews/ By-Any-Other-Name-Its-Still-Sweetener_UCM_437368_Article.jsp

7. Tyler G. Graham and Drew Ramsey, M.D., *The Happiness Diet* (New York: Rodale, 2011), 34.

8. U.S. Department of Agriculture, "Profiling Food Consumption in America," *USDA Agriculture Factbook.* http://www.usda.gov/factbook/chapter2.pdf

9. "Sugary Drinks and Obesity Fact Sheet," Harvard School of Public Health, 2013. http://www.hsph.harvard.edu/nutritionsource/sugary-drinks-fact-sheet/

10. S. W. Ng, et al., "Use of Caloric and Noncaloric Sweeteners in US Consumer Packaged Foods 2005 – 2009," University of North Carolina – Chapel Hill, PubMed.gov, November 2012. http://www.ncbi.nlm.nih.gov/pubmed/23102182

Robert Lustig, M.D., "Still Believe 'A Calorie Is a Calorie'?" *Huffington Post*, 27 February 2013. http://www.huffingtonpost.com/robert-lustig-md/sugar-toxic_b_2759564.html

11. Giovanni Targher, M.D., et al., "Risk of Cardiovascular Disease in Patients with Nonalcoholic Fatty Liver Disease," *New England Journal of Medicine*, 30 September 2010. http://www.nejm.org/doi/full/10.1056/NEJMra0912063

12. Françoise Clavel-Chapelon and Guy Fagherazzi, " 'Diet' Drinks Associated with Increased Risk of Type II Diabetes," *Inserm*, 7 February 2013. http://english.inserm.fr/press-area/diet-drinks-associated-with-increased-risk-of-type-ii-diabetes

13. American Autoimmune Related Diseases Association, "2011: The Cost Burden of Autoimmune Disease: The Latest Front in the War on Healthcare Spending." http://www.aarda.org/pdf/cbad.pdf

14. U.S. Department of Agriculture, "Profiling Food Consumption in America," *USDA Factbook*, 19. http://www.usda.gov/factbook/chapter2.pdf

15. Jonas F. Ludvigsson, M.D., Ph.D., et al., "Small-Intestinal Histopathology and Mortality Risk in Celiac Disease," *Journal of the American Medical Association*, 16 September 2009. http://jama.jamanetwork.com/article.aspx?articleid=184586

16. Kate Torgovnick, "The Single Best Way to Lose Weight," WebMD. http://www.webmd.com/diet/features/single-best-way-lose-weight

17. "Beating Mindless Eating," Cornell University Food and Brand Lab, 2011. http://foodpsychology.cornell.edu/research/beating-mindless-eating.html

18. Brian Wansink, "Bottomless Bowls: Why Visual Cues of Portion Size May Influence Intake," Cornell University Food and Brand Lab, 2011. http://foodpsychology.cornell.edu/research/beating-mindless-eating.html

19. A. Tchernof and J. P. Després, "Pathophysiology of Human Visceral Obesity: an Update," Centre Hospitalier Universitaire de Québec, PubMed.gov, January 2013. http://www.ncbi.nlm.nih.gov/pubmed/23303913

J. P. Block, et al., "Psychosocial Stress and Change in Weight among US Adults," Harvard Center for Population and Development Studies, PubMed.gov, 15 July 2009. http://www.ncbi.nlm.nih.gov/pubmed/19465744

20. "Soft Lighting and Music Cuts Calorie Intake 18 Percent," *Cornell Chronicle*, Cornell University, 29 August 2011. http://news.cornell.edu/stories/2012/08/soft-music-lighting-cuts-calories – 18-percent

21. "How Much Do You Spend on Food?" Gates Foundation, 2009. http://farm9
.staticflickr.com/8241/8456322351_03cb5f6e32_b.jpg

## CHAPTER 5: FITNESS

1. Megan Cochrane, "No Major Change in Americans' Exercise Habits in 2011,"
Gallup Wellbeing, 15 March 2012. http://www.gallup.com/poll/153251/no
-major-change-americans-exercise-habits – 2011.aspx

2. M. Babyak, J. A. Blumenthal, et al., "Exercise Treatment for Major Depression:
Maintenance of Therapeutic Benefit at 10 Months," *Psychosomatic Medicine,*
2000: 633 – 38.

   Jim Gavin, PhD, Daniel Seguin, and Madeleine McBrearty, PhD, "The Psychology of Exercise," IDEA Health & Fitness Association, February 2006. http://
www.ideafit.com/fitness-library/psychology-exercise – 1

3. Dan Britton, Jimmy Page, and Jon Gordon, *One Word That Will Change Your Life*
(Hoboken, NJ: Wiley and Sons, 2013).

4. William Sears, M.D., Peter Sears, M.D., and Sean Foy, *Dr. Sears' LEAN Kids*
(New York: New American Library, 2003).

5. "The Facts: What We Know about Sitting and Standing," JustStand.org, 2013.
http://www.juststand.org/TheFacts/tabid/816/language/en-US/Default.aspx

6. "Sitting May Increase Risk of Disease," *Science Daily,* 18 June 2013. www.science
daily.com/releases/2007/11/071119130734.htm

7. James Vlashos, "Is Sitting a Lethal Activity?" *The New York Times,* 14 April 2011.
http://www.nytimes.com/2011/04/17/magazine/mag – 17sitting-t.html?_r=0

8. Elin Ekblom-Bak, Mai-Lis Hellenius, and Bjorn Ekblom, "Are We Facing a New
Paradigm of Inactivity Physiology?" *British Journal of Sports Medicine,* February
2010. http://bjsm.bmj.com/content/44/12/834

9. James Vlashos, "Is Sitting a Lethal Activity?" *The New York Times,* 14 April 2011.
http://www.nytimes.com/2011/04/17/magazine/mag – 17sitting-t.html?_r=0

10. C. E. Garber, B. Blissmer, et al., "Quantity and quality of exercise for developing
and maintaining cardiorespiratory, musculoskeletal, and neuromotor fitness in
apparently healthy adults: Guidance for prescribing exercise." *Medicine & Science
in Sports & Exercise,* 2011: 1334 – 49.

    Len Kravitz, Ph.D., "Stretching – A Research Retrospective," IDEA Health &
Fitness Association, 2013. http://www.ideafit.com/fitness-library/stretching
-research-retrospective

11. S. L. Herman, et al., "Four-week dynamic stretching warm-up intervention elicits
longer-term performance benefits," *Journal of Strength and Conditioning Research,*
2008: 1286.

12. "Primetime Views: What Does the Phrase 'Young at Heart' Mean to You?" *Chicago Tribune,* 2013. http://www.chicagotribune.com/special/primetime/chi-primetime-ptviewsyoungheart – 071311,0,3417326.story

13. Stuart Brown, *Play: How It Shapes the Brain, Opens the Imagination, and Invigorates the Soul* (New York: Avery-Penguin Publishing, 2010).

14. Jean Lerche Davis, "Lose Weight with Morning Exercise," WebMD. http://www.webmd.com/fitness-exercise/features/lose-weight-with-morning-exercise
"Early Morning Exercise Is Best for Reducing Blood Pressure and Improving Sleep," Appalachian State University News, 13 June 2011. http://www.news.appstate.edu/2011/06/13/early-morning-exercise/

15. Bryant Stamford, Ph.D., "Cross-Training: Giving yourself a whole-body workout," *The Physician and Sportsmedicine,* September 1996.

16. Hayley E. Cutt, Matthew W. Knuiman, and Billie Giles-Corti, "Does Getting a Dog Increase Recreational Walking?" *International Journal of Behavioral Nutrition and Physical Activity,* 27 March 2008. http://www.ijbnpa.org/content/5/1/17

17. B. C. Irwin, et al., "Aerobic Exercise Is Promoted When Individual Performance Affects the Group," Michigan State University, PubMed.gov, October 2012. http://www.ncbi.nlm.nih.gov/pubmed/22576339

## CHAPTER 6: FOCUS

1. J. S. Cauffield and H. J. Forbes, "Dietary supplements used in the treatment of depression, anxiety, and sleep disorders," *Lippincotts Primary Care Practice,* 2009: 290 – 304.

2. "Teacher's Guide: Sleep — Information about Sleep," National Institutes of Health. http://science.education.nih.gov/supplements/nih3/sleep/guide/info-sleep.htm

3. M. Kivipelto, T. Ngandu, et al., "Obesity and vascular risk factors at midlife and the risk of dementia and Alzheimer disease," *Archives of Neurology,* October 2005: 1556 – 60. http://archneur.jamanetwork.com/article.aspx?articleid=789626

4. University of California – Davis, "High Blood Pressure Damages the Brain in Early Middle Age," *Science Daily,* 31 October 2012. http://www.sciencedaily.com/releases/2012/10/121031214240.htm

5. Y. Osher and R. H. Belmaker. "Omega – 3 fatty acids in depression: A review of three studies," *CNS Neuroscience & Therapeutics,* Summer 2009: 128 – 33.
K. C. Estes, B. T. Rose, et al., "Effects of omega 3 fatty acids on receptor tyrosine kinase and PLC activities in EMT6 cells," *Journal of Lipid Mediators and Cell Signaling,* 1999: 81 – 96.

6. "Stress in America Findings," American Psychological Association, 9 November 2010. http://www.apa.org/news/press/releases/stress/national-report.pdf

7. J. C. Pruessner, K. Dedovic, et al., "Stress regulation in the central nervous system: Evidence from structural and functional neuroimaging studies in human populations," *Psychoneuroendocrinology*, 9 April 2009.

   T. G. Dinan and J. F. Cryan, "Regulation of the stress response by the gut microbiota: Implications for psychoneuroendocrinology," *Psychoneuroendocrinology*, 4 April 2012.

8. "50 Common Signs and Symptoms of Stress," American Institute of Stress. http://www.stress.org/stress-effects/

9. Barbara Bradley Hagerty, "Prayer May Reshape Your Brain ... And Your Reality," NPR, 20 May 2009. http://www.npr.org/templates/story/story.php?storyId=104310443

   D. S. Khalsa, D. G. Amen, A. Newberg, et al., "Kirtan kriya meditation and high resolution brain SPECT imaging," accepted by *Nuclear Medicine Communications*, June 2010.

   Andrew Newberg, "The Effect of Meditation on the Brain Activity," AndrewNewberg.com, http://www.andrewnewberg.com/research.asp

10. Larry Dossey, *Healing Words: The Power of Prayer and the Practice of Medicine* (New York: HarperCollins, 1993).

    Dale A. Matthews with Connie Clark, *The Faith Factor: Proof of the Healing Power of Prayer* (New York: Penguin Books, 1999).

11. P. J. O'Connor, N. P. Pronk, et al., "Characteristics of adults who use prayer as an alternative therapy," *American Journal of Health Promotion*, May – June 2005: 369 – 75. http://www.ncbi.nlm.nih.gov/pubmed/15895540

12. H. G. Koenig, K. I. Pargament, and J. Nielsen, Department of Psychiatry, Duke University Medical Center, *Journal of Nervous and Mental Disorders*, September 1998: 513 – 21. http://www.ncbi.nlm.nih.gov/pubmed/9741556

13. David N. Elkins, "Spirituality," *Psychology Today*, 1 September 1999. http://www.psychologytoday.com/articles/199909/spirituality

14. M. P. Bennett, J. M. Zeller, et al., "The effect of mirthful laughter on stress and natural killer cell activity," *Alternative Therapies in Health and Medicine*, March – April 2003: 38 – 45. http://www.ncbi.nlm.nih.gov/pubmed/12652882

15. L. Stahre and T. Hallstrom, "A short-term cognitive group treatment program gives substantial weight reduction up to 18 months from the end of treatment," Eating and Weight Disorders, March 2005: 51 – 58. http://www.ncbi.nlm.nih.gov/pubmed/15943172

16. Ruth Streigel-Moore, G. Terence Wilson, et al., "Cognitive behavioral guided self-help for the treatment of recurrent binge eating," *Journal of Consulting and*

*Clinical Psychology,* June 2010. http://www.ncbi.nlm.nih.gov/pmc/articles/
PMC2880824/

17. "In Praise of Gratitude," *Harvard Mental Health Newsletter,* November 2011.
http://www.health.harvard.edu/newsletters/Harvard_Mental_Health_
Letter/2011/November/in-praise-of-gratitude

18. R. H. Pietrzak, J. Tsai, et al., "Successful Aging among Older Veterans in
the United States," *American Journal of Geriatric Psychiatry,* 26 March 2013.
http://www.ncbi.nlm.nih.gov/pubmed/23567414

19. R. A. Emmons and M. E. McCullough, "Counting blessings versus burdens:
an experimental investigation of gratitude and subjective well-being in daily
life," *Journal of Personality and Social Psychology,* February 2003.
http://www.ncbi.nlm.nih.gov/pubmed/12585811

20. Dr. Noelle C. Nelson, *The Power of Appreciation in Everyday Life* (Toronto:
Insomniac Press, 2006).

21. Martin E. Seligman, *Authentic Happiness* (New York: The Free Press, 2002).

22. A. Abdul-Rahman, C. D. Agardh, B. K. Siesjo, "Local cerebral blood flow in the
rat during severe hypoglycemia, and in the recovery period following glucose
injection," Acta Physiologica Scandinavian Physiological Society, 1980: 307–14.
http://www.ncbi.nlm.nih.gov/pubmed/?term=.+Local+cerebral+blood+flow+i
n+the+rat+during+severe+hypoglycemia%2C+and+in+the+recovery+period+f
ollowing+glucose+injection

## CHAPTER 7: FRIENDS

1. Steve Willis with Ken Walker, *Winning the Food Fight: Victory in the Physical and
Spiritual Battle for Good Food and a Healthy Lifestyle* (Ventura, CA: Regal, 2012).

2. Desiree Mohindra, "Non-communicable Diseases to Cost $47 Trillion by 2030,
New Study Released Today," World Economic Forum, 18 September 2011.
http://www.weforum.org/news/non-communicable-diseases-cost–47-trillion
–2030-new-study-released-today

3. Janelle Davis, "AAFP Foundation Global Director of Peers for Progress Outlines
Peer Support for Self-Management of Diabetes at Health Affairs Forum on
Diabetes," AAFP, 13 January 2012. http://www.aafp.org/media-center/releases
-statements/all/2012/peers-for-progress-self-management-diabetes.html

4. Tracy Kidder, *Mountains Beyond Mountains: The Quest of Dr. Paul Farmer,
a Man Who Would Cure the World* (New York: Random House, 2009).

5. Nicholas A. Christakis, M.D., Ph.D., M.P.H., and James H. Fowler, Ph.D.,
"The Spread of Obesity in a Large Social Network over 32 Years," *New England
Journal of Medicine,* 26 July 2007. http://www.nejm.org/doi/full/10.1056/
NEJMsa066082

6. Dan Buettner, "The Island Where People Forget to Die," *The New York Times,* 24 October 2012. http://www.nytimes.com/2012/10/28/magazine/the-island -where-people-forget-to-die.html?pagewanted=all

7. Dr. Dean Ornish, *Reversing Heart Disease* (New York: Ivy Books, 1996). D. Ornish, L. W. Scherwitz, et al., "Intensive lifestyle changes for reversal of coronary heart disease," *Journal of the American Medical Association,* 16 December 1998.

8. Dean Ornish, M.D., *Love and Survival* (New York: HarperCollins, 1998).

9. Walker Meade, "Loneliness takes toll on mental, physical health," *Herald-Tribune Health,* 14 February 2012. http://health.heraldtribune.com/2012/02/14/ loneliness-takes-toll-on-mental-physical-health/

10. Dr. Dean Ornish, "Q&A: How do loneliness and isolation affect our health?" *ShareCare.* http://www.sharecare.com/health/human-emotions/loneliness -isolation-affect-our-health;jsessionid=408BC4DAE90B4F7CBB0A7A71106 5DD76

11. Emma E. A. Cohen, Robin Ejsmond-Frey, et al., "Rowers' high: behavioural synchrony is correlated with elevated pain thresholds," *Biology Letters,* 15 September 2009. http://rsbl.royalsocietypublishing.org/content/early/ 2009/09/14/rsbl.2009.0670.full

## CHAPTER 8: LIVING THE LIFESTYLE

1. International Olympic Committee, "John Akhwari Fulfills His Commitment," *Teaching Values: An Olympic Education Toolkit* (Lausanne: International Olympic Committee, 2007), 111. http://www.olympic.org/Documents/OVEP_Toolkit/ OVEP_Toolkit_en.pdf

## CHAPTER 10: 40-DAY MEAL PLANS

1. Mark Hyman, M.D., *The Blood Sugar Solution: The UltraHealthy Program for Losing Weight, Preventing Disease, and Feeling Great Now!* (Boston: Little, Brown, 2012).

2. Mark Hyman, M.D., *The Blood Sugar Solution Cookbook: More Than 175 Ultra-Tasty Recipes for Total Health and Weight Loss* (Boston: Little, Brown, 2013).

# THE **DANIEL** PLAN

## The Daniel Plan Journal
### 40 Days to a Healthier Life

*Rick Warren*
*and The Daniel Plan Team*

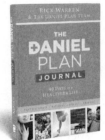

*The Daniel Plan Journal* is a practical and experiential tool filled with daily encouragement from Rick Warren and The Daniel Plan team. Scripture and inspirational quotes are also included. The journal was designed so users can record milestones related to all of The Daniel Plan Essentials: Faith, Food, Fitness, Focus, and Friends. This is an important element for those who want to maximize their potential to experience an all-around healthy lifestyle.

*Available in stores and online!*

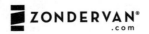

**ZONDERVAN®**
.com

## The Daniel Plan Cookbook

Healthy Eating for Life

*Rick Warren D.MIN.,*
*Daniel Amen M.D.,*
*and Mark Hyman M.D.*

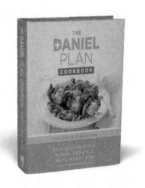

*The Daniel Plan Cookbook: Healthy Eating for Life* is a four-color cookbook filled with 100 delicious, Daniel Plan–approved recipes that offer an abundance of options to bring healthy cooking back into your kitchen. This eye-appealing cookbook is filled with easy-to-prepare, mouth-watering recipes. All the recipes are based on The Daniel Plan plate that emphasizes eating nutritionally packed whole foods. Choose from a variety of delicious options to create your weekly menu. Eating The Daniel Plan way not only is healthy and wholesome, but will boost your energy and kick-start your metabolism. The book includes practical tips from doctors, important food facts, and inspiration from the Daniel Plan signature chefs.

*Available in stores and online!*

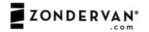

## The Daniel Plan
## Study Guide with DVD
## 40 Days to a Healthier Life

*Rick Warren D.MIN.,*
*Daniel Amen M.D.,*
*and Mark Hyman M.D.*

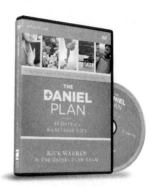

This six-session video-based, small group study from Rick Warren, Dr. Daniel Amen, and Dr. Mark Hyman is centered on five Essentials that will guarantee success in your health journey: faith, food, fitness, focus, and friends.

With assistance from medical and fitness experts, Pastor Rick Warren and thousands of people from his congregation started on a journey to transform their own lives. It's called The Daniel Plan, and it works for one simple reason: God designed your body to be healthy and vibrant, and he provided everything you need to thrive and live an abundant life.

This small group study is a vital component of The Daniel Plan because it bakes in the community aspect to its innovative approach to health. As Dr. Mark Hyman says, "Community is the medicine" for healthy living.

The Daniel Plan small group study teaches simple ways to incorporate healthy choices into your current lifestyle. This study guide includes Bible study, video discussion questions and notes, practical food and fitness tips to keep you on track each week, and much more.

### Session Titles
- **Faith:** Nurturing Your Soul
- **Food:** Enjoying God's Abundance
- **Fitness:** Strengthening Your Body
- **Focus:** Renewing Your Mind
- **Friends:** Encouraging Each Other
- **Living the Lifestyle**

## The Daniel Plan Mobile APP

The Daniel Plan App will be a dynamic app based on the cookbook/fitness book content but in a succinct, easy-to-understand-and-use format that provides wisdom and encouragement for each interaction. App will include a calorie counter, a feature for tracking progress on weight loss and 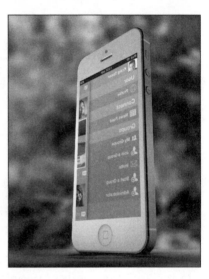 improving BMI (including the formula for calculating BMI), as well as a simple exercise log. Encouragement coupled with dietary facts and/or recipe ideas can be pushed to the user.

*Available in stores and online!*

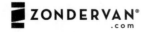

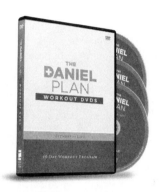
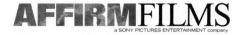

## Free Online Resources at
## www.zondervan.com

**Daily Bible Verses and Devotions:** Enrich your life with daily Bible verses or devotions that help you start every morning focused on God. Visit www.zondervan.com/newsletters.

**Free Email Publications:** Sign up for newsletters on Christian living, academic resources, church ministry, fiction, children's resources, and more. Visit www.zondervan.com/newsletters.

**Zondervan Bible Search:** Find and compare Bible passages in a variety of translations at www.zondervanbiblesearch.com.

**Other Benefits:** Register to receive online benefits like coupons and special offers, or to participate in research.

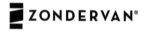

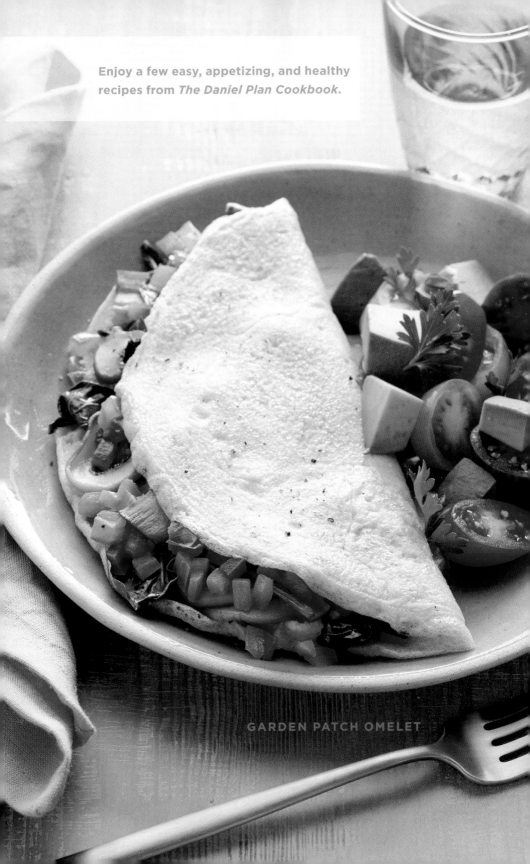

Enjoy a few easy, appetizing, and healthy recipes from *The Daniel Plan Cookbook*.

GARDEN PATCH OMELET

# Garden Patch Omelet

Filled with protein and fiber, vegetable omelets are a satisfying meal day or night.

**Serves 2**

3 eggs
¼ teaspoon Kosher or sea salt (optional)
Dash black pepper
2 teaspoons coconut oil, divided
¼ teaspoon minced garlic
1 cup baby spinach
¼ cup bell peppers (red, orange, yellow), diced
¼ cup red onion, diced
¼ cup tomato, diced
1 large mushroom, thinly sliced

1. In a bowl, whisk eggs with salt and pepper. Set aside.

2. Heat 1 teaspoon coconut oil over medium-high heat in a sauté or frying pan that has a lid. Add garlic, spinach, peppers, onion, tomato, and mushroom. Sauté until veggies are soft, about 3–5 minutes. Remove vegetables from pan. Set aside in a bowl.

3. Heat the remaining 1 teaspoon coconut oil in the pan. Pour the eggs in the pan evenly. Add in the veggies on top of the egg mixture, reduce heat to low, cover pan with lid. Cook for about 2 minutes. If the egg is still uncooked, cook for another minute uncovered. Fold the omelet in half.

4. Serve right away.

*The Daniel Plan Cookbook* includes more than 100 delicious, healthy recipes from breakfast to dessert.

# Lemony Dill Chicken Salad Pita

Enjoy a slight twist on a classic chicken salad. Try this as an open-face sandwich on gluten-free bread or rolled into a brown rice tortilla.

**Serves 4**

3 cups cooked chicken breast, chopped
4 small celery ribs, finely chopped
4 tablespoons red onion, finely chopped
1 generous tablespoon fresh dill, minced
4 tablespoons organic mayonnaise or Veganaise
A few squeezes of lemon juice
Salt and pepper to taste (or lemon pepper)
2 large whole wheat pitas, sliced in half
Red lettuce leaves
Sliced tomato (optional)

**1.** In a medium bowl, gently mix chicken, celery, onion, dill, mayonnaise, lemon juice, salt, and pepper.

**2.** Fill each pita half with a lettuce leaf, a slice or two of tomato, then a quarter of the chicken salad.

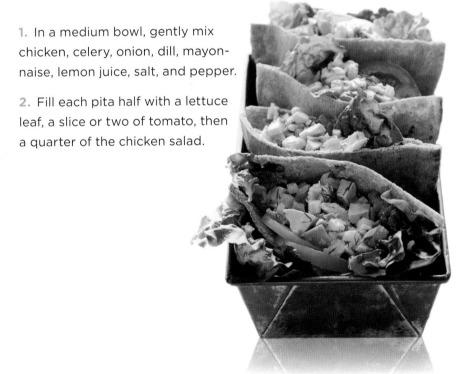

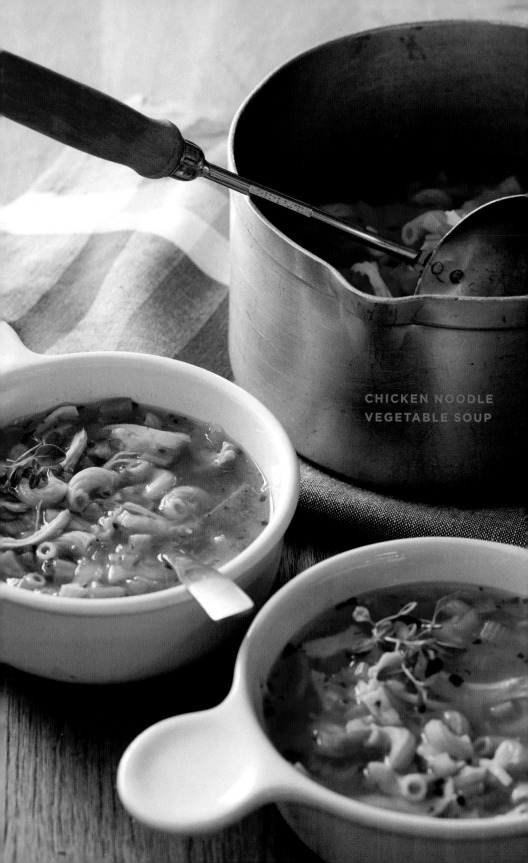

CHICKEN NOODLE
VEGETABLE SOUP

# Chicken Noodle Vegetable Soup

Classic and comforting, nothing is better than homemade chicken soup. It can be made in about an hour, even less if you use leftover roasted shredded chicken and precooked pasta. To make this gluten-free, use brown rice pasta.

**Serves 4–6**

2 tablespoons oil
3 ribs celery, finely chopped
2–3 carrots, finely chopped
1 medium onion, finely chopped
3 cloves garlic, minced
2 teaspoons fresh thyme, minced (or 3/4 teaspoon dried thyme)
1 bay leaf
Kosher or sea salt and pepper to taste
2 quarts (64 ounces) low-sodium chicken broth
1 large bone-in chicken breast (or shredded cooked chicken)
1 cup whole wheat or brown rice elbow pasta
1 tablespoon fresh parsley, chopped

1. Add oil to a large pot over medium heat. Turn the heat down to medium low and add the celery, carrots, and onion. Cook until the vegetables are soft and translucent, 12–15 minutes. Stir in the garlic, and cook another 30–60 seconds. Add thyme, bay leaf, salt, and pepper.

2. Remove skin and fat from chicken breast. Cut chicken breast crosswise through the bone into two pieces. Add the broth and the chicken breast to the pot. Bring to a boil, turn down to a simmer, and cook until chicken is cooked through, about 18 minutes.

3. Remove chicken from the pot. Add the pasta and simmer until pasta is tender. When chicken is cool enough to handle, shred the meat, and add back to the pot to warm.

4. Remove the bay leaf. Add parsley. Ladle into warm bowls to serve.

# Teriyaki Beef Stir Fry

One of the most popular Asian meals that we all enjoy is filled with broccoli, a high-fiber, high-nutrient veggie.

**Serves 4**

½ cup water
⅓ cup low-sodium soy or tamari sauce
2 tablespoons raw honey
¼ cup fresh orange juice (or pineapple)
4 garlic cloves, minced
1 tablespoon fresh ginger, cut into long thin strips
1 tablespoon fresh ginger, minced
1 pound flank steak, cut against the grain into thin strips
2 teaspoons coconut oil
4 cups broccoli florets
1 medium onion, chopped
1½ teaspoons cornstarch
2 cups brown rice

1. In a small bowl, combine the first six ingredients. Pour 1/2 cup of this mixture into a plastic bag; add beef. Seal bag, and turn to coat. Refrigerate for at least one hour. Cover and refrigerate remaining marinade.

2. Remove steak from bag, and discard marinade. In a large non-stick skillet or wok, stir-fry beef in oil for 2–3 minutes or until no longer pink. Remove and keep warm.

3. Add broccoli and onion to pan; stir-fry for 4 minutes, or until vegetables are tender.

4. Return beef to the pan. Whisk cornstarch and reserved marinade until smooth; stir into beef mixture. Bring to a boil; cook and stir until thickened, about 2 minutes. Serve over brown rice if desired.

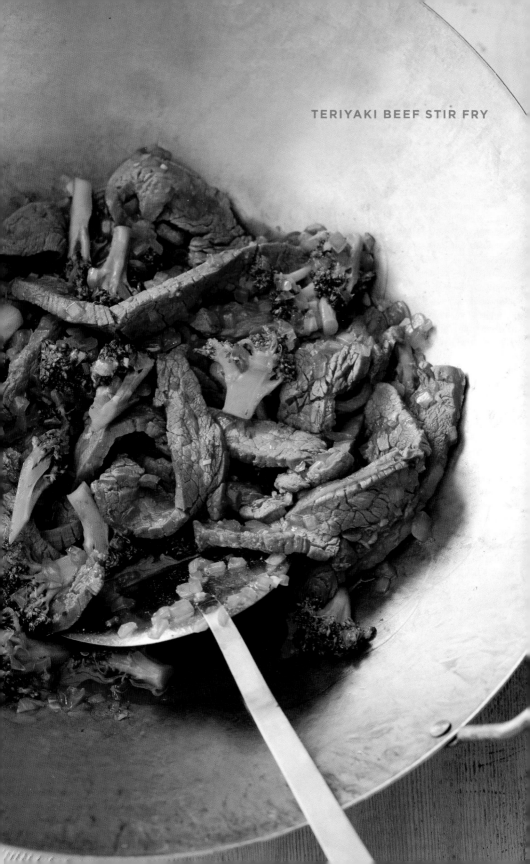

TERIYAKI BEEF STIR FRY

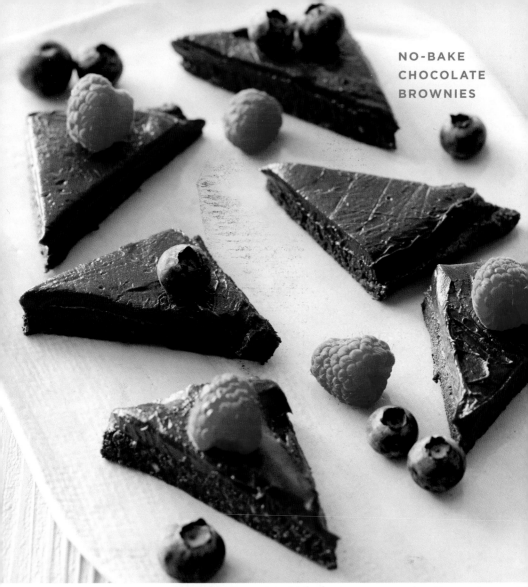

**NO-BAKE CHOCOLATE BROWNIES**

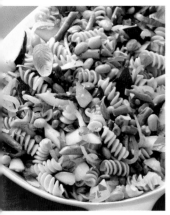

**PASTA PRIMAVERDE**

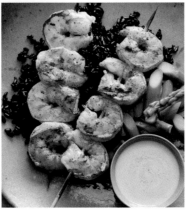

**GRILLED COCONUT LIME SHRIMP KABOBS**

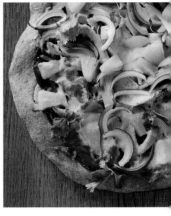

**BBQ CHICKEN PIZZA**